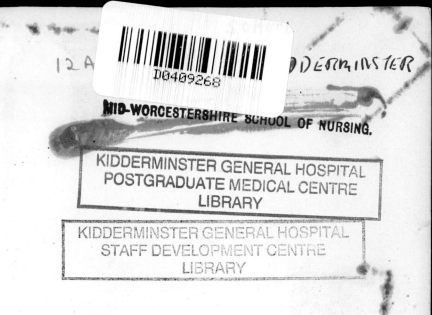

A Short History of Nursing

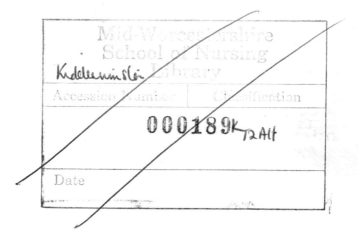

NURSING 42

A SHORT HISTORY
OF NURSING

★

W. R. BETT
M.R.C.S., L.R.C.P., F.R.S.L.,
F.S.A. Scot.

Illustrated by
MONA MOORE

FABER AND FABER LTD
24 Russell Square
London

First published in mcmlx
by Faber and Faber Limited
24 Russell Square London W.C.1
Printed in Great Britain by
Latimer Trend & Co Ltd Plymouth

To the 'Second Floor' of
the Lindo Wing
St. Mary's Hospital
for their skill, cheerfulness
and charm
when I was low in strength
and in spirit

Contents

Preface

While there are a number of excellent histories of nursing for the student nurse and the trained nurse to read or to consult, the girl who is thinking of taking up nursing as a career may find some of them too detailed for her liking, and she may complain that a good deal of the earlier material which they include is not strictly nursing history.

This book possesses the virtue of being short and of linking up, wherever possible, the past with the present. Of necessity, much has been left out, but this can be looked up in the more learned works listed in the bibliography.

For the reader to understand how the salaries mentioned in the various chapters compare with salaries today, she has to take into account not only the value of the money in terms of our money, but the buying power of it in our time. It is impossible to give accurate equivalent figures. In Shakespeare's time, for instance, money was probably worth about ten times what it is at present.

Miss Gertrude A. Ramsden, R.R.C., S.R.N., S.C.M., D.N., Research Organizer, Dan Mason Nursing Research Committee, National Florence Nightingale Memorial Committee, has very kindly read the

9

manuscript of my book and has helped me extensively with suggestions, criticisms, and facts, particularly relating to nursing today. It is a privilege to acknowledge her skilled and friendly help.

W. R. BETT.

London,
January, 1959.

Introduction

Any girl who has turned her thoughts towards nursing as a career will naturally want to know what type of girl took up nursing at various periods in history, and why; the duties she was expected to perform; the clothes she wore; the education, practical training, and salary she received; the social and professional status she enjoyed; the discipline to which she was subjected; and the rewards that came her way.

The story of nursing is very old. Its beginnings are lost in the mists of mythology and legend. The nurse was in existence before recorded history. Her healing touch is older than the oldest fragment of a medical manuscript that has ever been recovered. Her charity was tradition when the oldest of pyramids was being built. Throughout the ages, crimson with the blood of battle and aflame with cruelty and greed and lust, there were those who dressed the wounds of friend and foe, who fed the hungry, who clothed the naked, who comforted the sick, held out to them the hand of healing, and brought gladness to weary eyes. For woman has always been an instinctive nurse.

In that most readable book *White Caps: The Story of Nursing* (1946), Victor Robinson aptly describes the nurse as 'the mirror in which is reflected the position of woman through the ages'.

Amid the indescribable horrors of Scutari the infinite pity and the vindictive passion of The Lady-with-the-Lamp combined to lay the foundations of modern nursing. The girl of today becomes a trained nurse, not because she is unable to find other employment, but for humanity's sake. But before Florence Nightingale the nurse was a slave at first, then a domestic, then a nun who tended the sick for Christ's sake. Ignored by legislator and preceptor alike, she remained a pathetic paradox in history—indispensable, uneducated, untrained, without social status, without professional ethics.

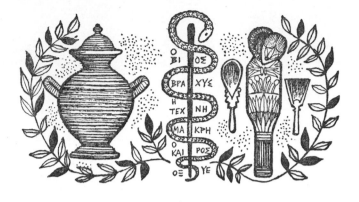

1

The Nurse in Ancient Times
Mere Glimpses of a Vague Figure

This is in many ways a disappointing chapter with which to start, for it is largely negative. But then our sources of information concerning nursing in ancient times are fragmentary. We can find a good deal recorded about medicine, hygiene, and even hospitals, but little mention of nurses and nursing. It is tempting to suggest—and this has been done quite often—that from the very beginnings of history the sick have always been nursed as a matter of course, but that historians have seldom thought it worthwhile to chronicle this necessary service. Is such an interpretation justified or is it historically more correct to assume that there were no professional nurses? But in that case, who did the everyday nursing?

In ancient Mesopotamia there are no records of nursing as such. The only reference to nursing among the old Egyptians is on an ostracon (an inscribed slab of limestone, No. 5634, from the reign of Ramesses II, about 1250 B.C.) in the British Museum, according to which certain labourers engaged in the construction of the tombs in the Valley of the Kings at Thebes, were excused from work because they were nursing sick members of their family. In the literature of ancient China it is impossible to identify any one with certainty as a nurse. Equally negative is the picture presented by the Hebrews. We know and respect them as accomplished masters in the art and science of hygiene. One of the greatest sanitarians who ever lived, Moses, when he was in charge of a huge camp of more than a million people, laid down scientific and almost modern rules for food inspection, disposal of excreta, and notification and quarantine of contagious diseases. Visiting the sick was the religious duty of all Israelite men and women. There were houses for strangers and houses for the sick—prototypes of the inn and the hospital—and separate houses for lepers, as witness 2 Kings xv. 5: 'And the Lord smote the king, so that he was a leper unto the day of his death, and dwelt in a several house.' Strangely, however, no records of nurses attending the inmates of the hospitals have been left by that enlightened people.

The early literature of the Indian peninsula is, however, more rewarding. Journeying through India, the Lord Buddha about 500 B.C. introduced the monastic system in the Orient and founded an order of nuns, about which, however, little is known.

The Nurse in Ancient Times

In the period 600 B.C.–A.D. 200 nursing had an important place in the treatment of the sick, though from the masculine gender commonly used in the Sanskrit references, it appears that female nurses were hardly ever employed. A number of ancient Hindu medical treatises contain accounts of hospitals and of 'attendants' (nurses), and detail the attributes of a good nurse. The *Caraka Samhita* lists knowledge of nursing, skill, affection for the patient, and cleanliness. The *Astanga Hridaya* insists that a nurse should be devoted to the patient, clean, clever in all duties, and intelligent. Other desirable qualities mentioned in the *Kasyapa* are good health, 'not given to disgust', and 'having control over the temper'. Absolute loyalty to the doctor in charge of the patient is demanded by the *Susruta Samhita*.

Nursing is classified as general nursing, midwifery, wet nursing, surgical nursing, and massage. The *Caraka Samhita* lays down that midwives be 'mothers of many children, sympathetic, constantly affectionate, of agreeable behaviour, resourceful, naturally kindhearted, cheerful, and tolerant of hardship'. Good reputation and close clipping of the nails are recommended as essential qualities by the *Susruta*. According to the *Susruta*,[1] the code of surgical nursing forbids the services of a female nurse. 'Not only that, even the sight of a woman is considered undesirable.'

Asoka, emperor of North India and disciple of the

[1] The reader is referred to an important article 'Nursing under ancient Indian systems (as described in Ayurvedic classics)' by K. K. Radhalaxmi and M. N. Rao, *Indian Journal of the History of Medicine*, 1956, 1, 36–40.

Buddha, around 225 B.C. built 18 hospitals (these were also medical schools), in which older women and men nursed the patients. He sent missionaries to Ceylon and converted the island to Buddhism. In Ceylon hospitals were endowed under royal munificence. King Dutugamunu, an important, but legendary figure in Singhalese history (*c.* 100–77 B.C.), erected several. Those attending the sick had to be proficient in cooking, in caring for bed patients, and in other nursing procedures, and it has been suggested that training schools for nurses must have been in existence then.

ANCIENT GREECE

What did the old Greek doctor do when he required the services of a nurse? If you think of ancient Greece as typically a man's world in which woman generally held a subordinate position, you will understand why Greek girls were not given any instruction in medicine or any training in nursing. This is all the more astonishing because the Greeks were the most intellectually gifted people in history. 'To one small people', wrote that brilliant jurist and classical scholar, Sir Henry Maine, 'it was given to create the principle of progress. That people was the Greek. Except the blind forces of nature nothing moves in this world which is not of Greek origin'. Yet that same people refused to admit that men and women could work together harmoniously, loyally, and in honoured partnership to safeguard health and to succour the sick.

In Greek mythology Zeus, omnipotent father of

gods and men, bestowed upon the earth goddess Hecate the role of the nursing mother of children, and ever since then every mother has instinctively played the role of nurse. While the nurse is frequently mentioned by Homer, the father of poetry, and by Herodotus, the father of history, Hippocrates, the father of medicine, ignores her completely in the *Corpus Hippocraticum*, the collection of 70 books attributed to him and to his school. Hippocrates (born about 460 B.C.), who created modern clinical medicine, who emancipated the art of healing from the shackles of superstition and magic, and who introduced accurate observation by the bedside, carefully described, and taught such common nursing procedures as making beds, sponging, bandaging, and preparing barley water. But who carried out these procedures? The Greek physicians were fully occupied, for malaria was endemic, typhus was epidemic, tuberculosis was prevalent. It is most unlikely that they found time for nursing duties. Often the burden of sick nursing fell on the patient's family, chiefly the wife or mother. There is an interesting passage, however, in the Hippocratic book *Decorum*, which suggests that in serious illness, when the doctor had to leave a patient who needed watching a medical student stayed in the sickroom:

'Let one of your pupils be left in charge, to carry out instructions without unpleasantness, and administer the treatment. Choose out those who have been already admitted into the mysteries of the art, so as to add anything necessary, and to give treatment with safety. He is there also to prevent those things escaping notice that happen in the intervals between visits. Never put a layman in charge of anything, otherwise if a mischance occur the blame will fall on you.'

Truly it has been said that the great Hippocrates laid the foundation of scientific medicine but, omitted the corner-stone of trained nursing.[1]

The nurse in ancient Greece was a wet nurse or nursemaid. In no sense was she the predecessor of the modern trained nurse.

ANCIENT ROME

The Romans with their genius for administration made great strides in public and private hygiene. Many of their achievements continue to astonish us. Their cities and towns had pure water supplies, aqueducts, and sewers. There were public baths and private baths in houses. There was even central heating. It was Christian monasticism that destroyed the cult of the Roman bath, but more about this in the next chapter. Military surgeons were attached to the Roman armies, and remains of military hospitals have been dug up in various parts of Europe. Trained slaves served as hospital attendants and worked under the doctors' orders. In the pre-Christian days there were no female nurses.

---

[1] There was no lack of midwives, known as *omphalotomai* (navel-cutters), but they were not trained women and did not work in co-operation with the doctors.

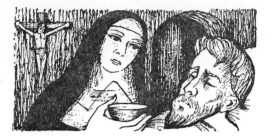

2

The Nun Becomes a Nurse

For the first time, woman dedicating her life to nursing the sick enters our story. It is with the advent and rise of Christian monasticism that we meet her tending patients in hospital, for Christ's sake.

Christian monasticism may be said to have begun in the year A.D. 305, when St. Anthony, surnamed the Great, built the first monastery near Aphroditopolis—the modern Atfih—on the right bank of the Nile. Born at Koma in Upper Egypt, he renounced the world at the age of twenty and became one of the earliest Christian hermits. Another Egyptian, St. Pachomius (A.D. 292–346), established nine monasteries of men, and the first nunnery at Tabennisi near Dendera. His was the first Christian religious order, the Pachomian monks.

A Greek, St. Basil, also surnamed the Great, in 370, when bishop of Caesarea in Cappadocia, Asia

Minor, built outside the city gates a hospital town, known after him as the Basileas. Its foundation is believed to have been inspired by the dire needs of the many lepers in Asia Minor and, more directly, by the great famine of 368. The most amazing creation in the annals of early hospitals, the Basileas provided separate buildings for lepers; homes for the aged, for orphans, for cripples, for the mentally afflicted; a rehabilitation centre; accommodation for the convalescent; and private residences for the medical and nursing staff. A capable administrator and a man of vision and infinite charity, whose footsteps were dogged by constant ill health, St. Basil took an enlightened interest in nursing, which he described as the most noble of all professions. He had a beautiful and pious sister, Macrina, a deaconess, whom he appointed superintendent of nurses.

If only we knew something of the training of monastic nurses and of the principles and practice of nursing in those days! Unhappily we know next to nothing. While there were many advances, there were also many retrograde steps. It was, above all, the oriental idea of 'sickness and sin' that was responsible for putting back the clock of medical progress. Sickness in the early days of Christianity was regarded as divine in origin, sent into this world to test the faith of the good and to punish the evil. Its treatment, therefore, also had to be theological. No longer did the profession of medicine subscribe to the Hippocratic doctrine of the natural causation of disease. No longer did it believe in the healing power of Nature. Medicine had ceased to be a science. Nursing, too, was theological, not medical, born not of science, but of the gospel of charity and mercy and love. It is no exaggeration to say that the nurse's primary duty was not to nurse a sick body back to health, but to prepare the immortal soul within that mortal body to meet its Maker. But who can doubt that the calmness of her presence, the soft touch of her hand, the gentleness of her voice, brought comfort and peace and hope to many a troubled and weary heart: Abide with us: for it is toward evening, and the day is far spent.

Nursing without bathing! The very thought seems incredible to us today. One's pen almost revolts at recording it. Yet it is an historic fact that monastic nursing forbade the use of the bath which had almost become a ritual to the Romans of old. The foundation of this anachronism was the implicit belief that concern for the cleanliness and comfort of the body and its garments spelled impurity of the soul, that whoever was once washed in the blood of Christ need not wash again.

The first free hospital (*nosocomion*) in Rome, supported by Christians, was founded in 390 by Fabiola, a beautiful and exceedingly wealthy patrician lady. Her history is a strange one. She had married a depraved husband, whom she divorced. A second marriage likewise proved to be a tragic failure. She then embraced Christianity and, lavishing her immense fortune on the poor and sick, she threw herself, body and soul, into a life of service to them. When she died, all Rome followed her to her grave. On her death St. Jerome wrote a remarkable letter which Victor Robinson calls 'the first literary document in the history of nursing':

'She founded a hospital and gathered into it sufferers from the streets, giving their poor bodies worn with sickness and hunger all a nurse's care. Need I describe here the diverse troubles from which human beings suffer, the maimed noses, the lost eyes, the scorched feet, the leprous arms, the swollen bellies, the shrunken thighs, the dropsical legs, and the diseased flesh alive with hungry worms? How often did she carry on her own shoulders poor filthy wretches tortured by epilepsy! How often did she wash away the purulent matter from wounds which others could not even endure to look upon! She gave food with her own hand, and even when a man was but a breathing corpse, she would moisten his lips with drops of water.'

Fabiola had a great friend, a learned and fabulously rich noble lady named Paula, who also became a Christian. Paula left Rome about 385 and sailed for Palestine where she built hospitals for the sick on the road to Bethlehem, and a monastery at Bethlehem itself. She established a hospital convent for women at Jerusalem. Paula is one of the most important, but tantalizingly elusive, figures in the early chronicles of nursing. She has been described as one of the first trained nurses in history. But who trained her we shall never know.

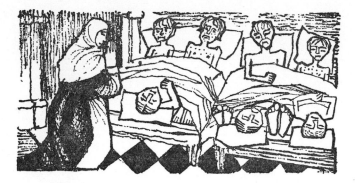

3

The Middle Ages
A Millennium of Intellectual Darkness

The Middle Ages is a conventional term applied to a period in western European history of roughly a thousand years—A.D. 500 to 1500. More precisely, the Middle Ages may be said to have begun in 476, when the last of the nominal rulers of Imperial Rome, Romulus Augustulus, was dethroned by the Teutonic chief Odoacer (Ottokar), who established a German kingdom on Italian soil. The Middle Ages ended, according to many historians, in 1453 with the capture of Constantinople by the Turks and with the beginning of the Renaissance.

A long and generally barren period over which broods the shadow of the uselessness of human endeavour; a period, however, when the first 'career'

23

outside marriage was thrown open to woman—the career of convent life. Nowhere else could she obtain an 'education', however narrow and bigoted such education may appear to us today.

This millennium of intellectual darkness is illuminated by such shining figures as St. Benedict, St. Francis and Clara of Assisi, St. Catherine of Siena; it is made memorable by the formulation of humane, wise, and at times quite modern nursing rules; it becomes historically important because of the foundation of the various nursing orders.

ST. BENEDICT AND HIS RULE

Patriarch of western monasticism, St. Benedict of Nursia in Italy (*c.* 480–543) in 529 built a monastery at Monte Cassino and inaugurated the Benedictine order of monks (the Black Monks). Some three years before his death, of a fever contracted while nursing the poor, he drew up the Benedictine rule which is eloquent of his humanity, his spiritual wisdom, and his essential simplicity: it laid down that the sick must be 'ministered unto as though indeed it were unto Christ'.

There were three main classes of nursing orders: the military or Knights Hospitallers, to be dealt with in the chapter 'The Nurse Goes to War'; the secular orders which originated outside the Church, but were under its protection; and the regular orders, e.g. The Augustinian Sisters of the Hôtel-Dieu in Paris.

At one time a public 'infirmarium' or sick bay formed part of a monastery, being administered by the abbot. Its nurses were of two types: professional nurses who searched for and admitted those who were sick, and pious women who worked out their own salvation by ministering to the patients. Anxious to be truly acceptable unto the Lord, they often did hygienically foolish things such as lovingly kissing the unwashed feet of beggars.

It was not until the twelfth century that homes for the aged and the destitute poor were separated from hospitals for the sick. The latter, however, continued to belong to the Church, and they remained ecclesiastical, not medical institutions.

THE CLOISTERED NUN

The story of nursing in one of the oldest hospitals on the continent of Europe, the Hôtel-Dieu of Paris, which was founded in the year 650, forms one of the most amazing and most pathetic sections in our book. It is the story of women forsaking the outer world for twelve unbroken centuries to lead a cloistered existence and finally to die within the narrow walls of one institution; heeding not the miracle of spring, the gentle sorrow of autumn; oblivious of the blessings of peace, of the terror of war, of the spectre of famine and pestilence stalking the land. Creatures of a half-world between the quick and the dead, they paced the twenty-five wards and the endless gloomy corridors, night and day, their eyes shining with spiritual exaltation. But spiritual exaltation went hand in hand with intellectual atrophy.

You must think of these Augustinian nuns nursing the sick, knowing little of the structure of the human body and even less of its functions. To their narrow outlook seeking knowledge of physiology was improper, and curiosity about things anatomical was sinful. There was no preliminary training school for the student nurse. We have no records of any lectures ever being given. Each novice was placed in the individual care of a sister for personal tuition, but what this personal tuition was we do not know.

During her period of probation, which was seldom less than twelve years, the nurse was known first as *fille en approbation*; she then wore a white robe and became *fille blanche*; and finally she received the hood of *fille à chaperon*.

What were the duties of these White Daughters of Christ? They had to admit the sick and nurse them empirically, for a diagnosis was rarely made. The patient entering the hospital made his confession, gave up all his clothes and, wearing nothing but a nightcap, was put to bed with other patients. In times of pestilence when the wards were crowded, as many as six patients shared one bed, lying feet opposite faces. The beds were huge, high, far too heavy to move, and so close together that they could not be scrubbed. The straw in the mattresses was changed three times a year. There were bed curtains, feather pillows, sheets, and grey cloth quilts lined with the mixed fur of sheep, dogs, cats, squirrels, and foxes.

The nuns were responsible also for the cooking and the laundering. The only laundry was the Seine outside the hospital gates. Fully habited, the novices had to wade into the river. In winter they broke the ice and stood for hours in the water, frozen to their knees. The patients also had to share the discomforts of this primitive system, for the wet clothes and sheets were hung in the unventilated wards to dry.

Thus twelve bleak centuries slowly dragged themselves by. In the year 1908 the Augustinian nuns were expelled from the Hôtel-Dieu. Some, having realized like Rip van Winkle of old, that neither for themselves nor for others had Time stood still, later returned to the hospital from exile with the torch of the new learning and the healing hand of the trained nurse. Others, incapable of resigning themselves to the complete transformation of all values in their lives, never entered the hospital again.

THE DARK AGES OF NURSING IN ENGLAND

Medieval piety in England founded many famous hospitals and institutions for the sick, the aged, the destitute, and the insane, and special houses for lepers. A Saxon hospital at St. Albans is mentioned as early as 794. St. Peter's at York was built in 937. A home for lepers at Rochester is believed to have been in existence before 1100. St. Bartholomew's Hospital in London was founded by Rahere in 1123. St. Oswald's at Worcester dates back to before 1268.

Then came the Reformation, that violent revolution in which northern Europe threw off the papal supremacy of Rome and in whose name stupid blunders and infamous crimes were committed. Henry VIII broke with the Pope in 1534. Two years later the short-sighted and disastrous Dissolution of the Monasteries closed all the houses of

Christian philanthropy—the only places in England where a woman with a vocation for nursing could spend her life. The English religious orders were dispersed, and no organizations were provided to take their place. All the nuns in the country were scattered like autumn leaves, with the notable exception of the women of the Order of St. Bridget of Sweden, who had built a wealthy nunnery at Syon House near Isleworth on the Thames and who now migrated to the Netherlands in an unbroken group. These nuns, by the way, had a remarkable set of rules governing conventual behaviour and the treatment of the sick, with detailed instructions on changing the beds, feeding the patients, and administering medicines. They were told not to be impatient or angry with those of their charges suffering from 'the flux' or 'the frenzy', 'for there be some sickness vexing the sick so greatly and provoking them to ire that the matter drawn up to the brain alienates the mind'. These are probably the earliest instructions on psychiatric nursing.

The monasteries were restored in 1554, but again suppressed five years later, when all monastic possessions were vested in the Crown. St. Bartholomew's Hospital was refounded in 1544 by Henry VIII who, however, two years afterwards once again took over its possession. The king's physicians were in the habit of saying that the only means of persuading him to listen to reason was to have him fall ill! It was on his death-bed in 1547 that Henry founded the Royal Hospitals—St. Bartholomew's and St. Thomas's.

It is interesting to note the change in social status

of the women nursing the sick in the refounded hospitals: no longer did they come from old and wealthy families, but from the poor districts of Smithfield and Southwark.

ST. FRANCIS AND ST. CLARA OF ASSISI

Let us go to Italy next to meet three important people in the history of medieval nursing.

The son of a rich cloth-merchant, Francesco Bernadone (1182–1226)—you know him better as St. Francis of Assisi—gave up the world, founded the Franciscan (First) Order of the Grey Friars, and became nursing missionary to the social outcasts, the lepers. His young disciple Clara of Assisi he installed in the convent of San Damiano whose abbess she remained for forty years. In 1212 St. Clara established the (Second) Order of the Franciscan nuns known as Poor Clares or Poor Clarisses, whose duties included nursing the sick and attending to lepers in little mud huts grouped around the convent. One of the most tragic cases they had to nurse at San Damiano was one of consumption: a pale gaunt man with cadaverous face and burning eyes; doubly tragic—because he died so young, yet prematurely old, at the age of 44—and because he was the founder and sustainer of their faith. St. Francis also created a Third Order, the Tertiaries, a religious association of lay men and women who led ordinary lives in the world.

ST. CATHERINE OF SIENA, PATRONESS OF NURSING

One of the most remarkable women in the annals

of medieval nursing is Catherine Benincasa of Siena (1347–80), who early in life joined the Tertiaries of St. Dominic. Her energy, vitality, and humanity were such that she made a name for herself as nurse, mystic, preacher, and reformer. At the hospital of Santa Maria della Scala opposite the cathedral of Siena she ministered to the repulsive victims of leprosy, advanced cancer, and bubonic plague, and organized parties of stretcher-bearers to convey the sick to the wards. Like the famous Lady-with-the-Lamp—the heroine of our next chapter—she carried a little lamp when she visited the hospital at night.

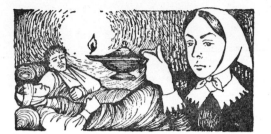

4

Florence Nightingale, Creator of Modern Nursing: Nursing Becomes a Profession

How shall we portray the heroine of this chapter? Shall we redraw the legendary figure of the saintly Lady with the Lamp, whose very shadow on the wall the soldier blessed as it passed his couch? Shall we sketch the pale, thin, angular woman with the haughty eyes and the bitter mouth, bullying, 'raging insatiably', a mistress of intrigue? Shall we paint the life-long neurotic, the invalid who spent nearly half a century in one room, eating her meals alone, seeing visitors by special appointment; whose infirmities shielded her from her opponents who did not wish to hurt a sick woman's feelings? The canvas is vast, the picture is composite, the portrait has its lights and its shades.

The second daughter of William and Fanny Nightingale was born on 12th May 1820 at Florence in Italy, and on July 4th was baptized Florence. Her

sister was born a year earlier at Naples, the ancient
Greek Parthenope, from which she took her unusual
Christian name Parthenope, shortened to Parthe, or
Pop. There were no other children. The family was
rich, owning two beautiful estates, Lea Hurst in
Derbyshire and Embley Park in Hampshire on the
edge of the New Forest. It had little to do except
attend or throw elaborate parties, go to church, and
travel abroad.

While such a life suited the parents and their
elder daughter, it certainly did not suit Florence. She
was different from other well-bred English children:
shy, moody, obstinate, introspective, dreamy, rebel-
liously discontent with being busy only with idle-
ness. She was unhappy, and her family could not
understand why. She was not quite seventeen when,
on 7th February 1837, she had a strange mystical
experience which she interpreted to be a call from
God to His Service. Some seven years later she first
realized that she was called to nurse the sick, but
when she asked for permission to work for a few
months as a nurse at Salisbury Hospital where a
friend of the Nightingales was on the medical staff,
her family was profoundly shocked. She was reminded that no nice girl ever left home except to get
married, and that nurses were servants with whom
no one would associate. Inevitably the chasm of mis-
understanding between the unhappy girl and her
family became wider and wider.

It is interesting to observe that in the autumn of
1842 Florence was told by the Prussian Ambassador
in London of Pastor Theodore Fliedner and his
wife, who in 1833 had equipped a summer house in

their back-garden on the Rhine with a bed and a chair as a refuge for a destitute discharged prisoner. This was the humble nucleus of the famous Kaiserswerth Institute for Protestant Deaconesses, opened in 1851, and comprising a hospital with 100 beds, a school for infants, an orphan asylum, and a training establishment for nurses.

But Florence was not interested. Her hour was not yet. Her unhappiness reached breaking point when in 1849 one of the social lions of the day, Richard Monckton Milnes (afterwards Baron Houghton of Great Houghton), who was deeply in love with her, asked for her hand in marriage. There is no doubt that she, too, was genuinely fond of him, yet she turned him down, for she was afraid that as his wife she would have nothing else to do but supervise the arrangement of dinner parties.

We shall see later how this deliberate repression of the sex-instinct was to play havoc with her nervous system. During the months that followed, physically and mentally fatigued, subject to repeated fainting attacks, and feeling unutterably frustrated, she snatched contentedness at odd hours by studying reports of sanitary commissions, watching surgical operations, and visiting slums. In 1851 she spent three short months with the German peasant girls at the Kaiserswerth Institute, where work was hard and life spartan.

There is the astonishing and revealing story of how Parthe accompanied Florence to the door of the Institute on her arrival there. In a fit of renouncement Florence offered her bracelets to her sister. But Parthe threw them back in a rage. Florence collapsed in a dead faint—the beginning, as she recorded, of her grave illness. Though Kaiserswerth had whetted her appetite for nursing, she would not admit that she had been trained there, for she described the nursing as 'nil', the hygiene as 'horrible'. She became a novice in a convent school at Rome, she worked with the Sisters of Saint Vincent de Paul in Paris. Without nursing her life was empty and useless.

Florence Nightingale had passed her 33rd birthday before her parents allowed her to accept her first position, that of superintendent of the Establishment for Gentlewomen during Illness at No. 1 Upper Harley Street, from 12th August 1853—October 1854. There at long last she was not only content, she was happy, being triumphantly aware of her great powers of administration. There also she learnt a most valuable lesson, that, in order to manage an institution successfully, one must instil in the governing body unconscious subservience to oneself.

In August 1854 a ghastly epidemic of cholera swept London. Florence Nightingale, working day and night, undertook at The Middlesex Hospital 'the superintendence of the cholera patients . . . brought in every half hour from the Soho district, Broad Street, etcetera'. It was in those terrible days that she gained much of the experience that was to be so useful to her at Scutari. She was convinced that cholera was not 'infectious from person to person'. Of all those in the hospital who came in contact with the disease only one nurse died of cholera.

THE CRIMEAN WAR

Then the Crimean War began, and out of its nightmare rose Florence Nightingale the Reformer and the profession of nursing. Never in her history had England drifted into a war with so little preparation. Never had so many of her soldiers perished because of entangling red tape, tragically obsolete administration, 'killed by antiquated imbecility'.

In a letter dated 15th October 1854, the Secretary-at-War, Sidney Herbert, first Baron Herbert of Lea, strikingly handsome and ahead of his time as a sanitarian, requested Florence Nightingale to go to Scutari with the Government's sanction and at the Government's expense. Her letter offering her services crossed his in the post.

It seems almost incredible to us today to read of the difficulties she had in recruiting 38 suitable nurses for this expedition. She finally selected 5 White Nuns, 5 Bermondsey Nuns, 6 nurses from St. John's House, 8 Anglican sisters, and 14 hospital nurses. Several of these, she realized only too well, were obvious misfits.

The uniform selected was ugly and unbecoming, consisting of a grey tweed dress, called a 'wrapper', a grey worsted jacket, plain white cap, short woollen cloak, and a 'frightful' holland scarf on which 'Scutari Hospital' was embroidered in red. Time did not permit to fit individual wearers.

The party left London Bridge on 21st October 1854 and travelled via Boulogne and Paris to Marseilles. From Marseilles, they continued their voyage to Constantinople in a fast mail boat, the *Vectis*, infested with huge cockroaches. A bad sailor, Florence was prostrated with seasickness. When they landed at Constantinople on November 3rd, there greeted their incredulous eyes on the opposite shore their new home—an enormous Turkish barrack hospital. When they reached it it proved to have vast echoing corridors, four miles of beds, floors of broken tiles, walls steaming damp, a courtyard in the centre—a veritable sea of mud littered with refuse. The hospital was built over a huge concealed Turkish sewer which had no outward ventilation. The drains were broken. The stench was indescribable. The patients were piled up in the corridors on unwashed filthy floors crawling with vermin. There were no pillows or blankets; no water, no pail to carry water; no soap, towels, combs, or brushes. Suppurating wounds were not dressed; fractured bones were not set.

It was in this inferno of filth and horror and misery that Florence Nightingale, then in her 35th year, single-handed and 'raging insatiably'—to use the Homeric phrase applied to her by the Master of Balliol—organized a highly efficient hospital and sanitary system which made the after-treatment of surgical operations possible to contemplate, and laid the foundation stone of modern nursing. But her most deadly enemies were not starvation, exposure, frostbite, gangrene, scurvy, dysentery, erysipelas, typhus, cholera. Her worst and most persistent foe was red tape.

Vast quantities of material sent from England for the soldiers at Scutari were allowed to rot in the seaport of Varna on the western shore of the Black Sea.

Vast quantities were buried and forgotten beneath munitions, voyaging uselessly backwards and forwards across the waters of the Black Sea until they were discovered by sheer accident. And when finally a shipment did arrive, it had to await inspection by a leisurely Board of Survey. At one time more than a thousand patients suffered from acute diarrhoea, and there were only twenty chamber pots. The privies had been allowed to become useless. Florence Nightingale had a large sum of money at her disposal—more than £30,000, and the first things she bought were 200 hard scrubbing brushes and sacking for washing the floors. Some of her nurses she had to send home because they were drunk while on duty, stole comforts intended for the patients, and committed immoral acts with the orderlies.

THE NIGHTINGALE SCHOOL

Already a heroine of the nation, Florence Nightingale returned to England to win even greater glory. By national subscription a Nightingale Fund of £44,000 was collected, which was used to establish a training school for nurses. In June 1860, after much careful planning, the first fifteen probationers were admitted for one year's training to the Nightingale School at St. Thomas's Hospital, the Fund paying their salaries and the Hospital providing working facilities. At the completion of one year the nurses joined the hospital staff for a further two years' experience. By the innovation of a prescribed period of training nursing became a respectable profession and an independent career for women whose emancipation was recognized. Nightingale nurses were soon in great demand. Many hospitals at home and abroad during the next decade asked Miss Nightingale for trainees from her school to join their staff so that they might organize training schools and improve the standard of nursing. Miss Nightingale's revolutionary innovation in training nurses was that under her system the control of the nurses was vested in the matron who must herself be a trained nurse. Her school, however, remained unique because of the Nightingale Fund. No other hospital in this country had separate financial resources for nurse training.

It is strange to record that to Miss Nightingale registration was complete and utter anathema. Nursing, she felt, was a sacred calling which could not be organized like a trade union; examinations, however practical, left out the question of a nurse's character. And so powerful was her influence for good and for evil, that as long as she lived and for some years after her death, it was impossible for a nurse in Britain to become registered.

Florence Nightingale's *Notes on Nursing* was published in 1859—a long time ago. But do read it. It is well worth reading. 'That classical compendium of the besetting sins of the sisterhood, drawn up with the detailed acrimony, the vindictive relish, of a Swift', Lytton Strachey described it. Be that as it may, this little book refuses to be dated: it is full of charm and full of witty sayings.

The long remainder of Florence Nightingale's life often makes sad reading. As she became more mellow and more benevolent in character, her physical appearance altered. The pale emaciated woman was gradually transformed into a stout old lady with a large, round, good-humoured face. She had founded her training school in 1860. She died in her sleep on 13th August 1910, at the ripe old age of 90. There was a final tragic period of obese senility, but the intervening fifty years beneath their cloak of invalidism were alive with incessant productive toil and dynamic energy.

When she had completed the report of the Commission reforming the Army Medical Services in August 1857, Miss Nightingale collapsed, her pulse became rapid, and from then until her death she lived in bed or on a couch. What, then, was the nature of invalidity? There was no organic disease, she was not paralysed, she lived to see many of her younger friends go before her into the grave. Though she constantly referred to herself as a weak person who was incapable of making any great or sustained effort, which would result in palpitations, rapid breathing, faintness, and pain, we know that she found no difficulty in working at anything that really interested her. Sir Zachary Cope in his scholarly and fascinating essay[1] 'Miss Florence Nightingale and the Doctors' (*Proceedings of the Royal Society of Medicine, Section of the History of Medicine*, 1956, 49, 907–14) diagnoses her condition to be a neurosis. His article repays careful study, for it provides food for thought, material for reflection.

In addition to being the creator of modern nurs-

[1] Published in book form, *Florence Nightingale and the Doctors* (London: Museum Press Ltd., 1958).

ing, Florence Nightingale has many other reforms to her credit. Her contributions to improvements in hospital buildings, sanitation, and the Army Medical Services, and her pioneer work in statistics makes her one of the greatest Victorians.

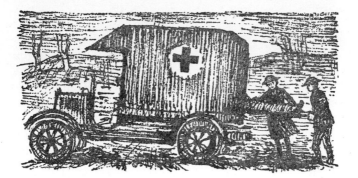

5

The Nurse Goes to War

The story of the military nursing orders is inseparably interwoven with that of the Crusades, those quixotic, disastrous expeditions which drained the blood of many nations; expeditions which were at the same time religious pilgrimages, military adventures, and paranoiac means of escape from the monotony of life.

Back in the seventh century Palestine had been torn from the Byzantine Empire by the Moslems who, being tolerant people, permitted pilgrims from Europe to continue visiting the Holy Places. In 1076 the Seljukian Turks, descendants of the Ghuz chieftain Seljuk and fervent champions of Islam, overran the country and persecuted the Christians. In the memorable and fatal year 1095 hundreds of thousands of men and women of all ages from every corner of the Continent rose to the clarion call of

Pope Urban II to form an army, march upon Jerusalem, and rescue the Holy Land from the domination of the Infidels. While many went in a dedicated frame of mind, some were criminals running away from justice; some were debtors escaping from their creditors; some were hysterical psychopaths; some were adventurers dreaming of renown and of the rich spoils of the East. If they died on active service, they could hope for the crown of martyrdom.

Their battle cry was *Deus vult* (it is the will of God), their symbol the Cross; hence the term Crusades. They could not wait to organize themselves into a properly equipped army. Under the fanatical leadership of Peter de Acheris 'the Hermit', mounted on his mule, these undisciplined hordes marched towards the Holy City. Their provisions were tragically scant, for they had blind faith in a God who had fed the hungry children of Israel with manna in the wilderness. Thousands perished miserably on the way, to feed the jackals and the vultures. Those who survived were scattered by the enemy.

The next expedition, however, was carefully organized and in 1099 successfully stormed the Holy City. The establishment of a Christian Kingdom in Jerusalem which existed for 87 years, saw the growth of the military nursing orders or Knights Hospitallers. The first to take the stage was the Order of the Hospital of St. John of Jerusalem (known later as the Knights of Rhodes and the Sovereign Order of the Knights of Malta). This Order had been 'instituted' as a charitable brotherhood in 1087 by a certain Gerard or Gerald, head of the hospital dedicated to St. John the Baptist, to relieve pilgrims.

The Nurse Goes to War

The original purpose of the Nursing Order of St. John was solely to bring in the wounded and to work in the hospitals; hence the term Hospitallers.

At a later stage the Knights were compelled to establish a fighting branch to defend the wounded while they were carried into hospital, and also to defend the pilgrims when attacked. Gerard was succeeded as Grand Master in 1120 by Raymond du Puy, who gave the Order the Augustinian Rule and divided it into three classes: priests, knights, and *frères sergents*, or serving brothers, who did the actual nursing. A very rich Order, it equipped its own hospitals in Jerusalem—splendid institutions in which the patients were lovingly cared for and supplied with plentiful good food. The hospital of St. John the Almoner for men was associated with the church of Santa Maria della Latina, and in the middle of the twelfth century had accommodation for 2,000 patients.

The female branch of the Order is as old as the male. As early as the first Crusade, a Roman lady named Agnes founded in Jerusalem the hospital of Mary Magdalene for women. The sisters lived under the mother superior, but obeyed the rules of St. John's Brothers. Until 1187, when they fled to Europe, they devoted themselves to prayer and to sick-nursing; thereafter they became a purely contemplative Order. In the beginning they wore garments resembling those of the Knights Hospitallers: red with an octagonal white cross, but after the fall of Rhodes they changed to black as a token of grief.

When Jerusalem was recaptured by Saladin, Sultan of Egypt in October 1187, the Knights lost their hospitals, and when in May 1291 Acre, the last hope of the Christians in the Holy Land fell into enemy hands, they were forced to abandon all their remaining possessions in the country. The flower of Christian chivalry was slain or captured. A small remnant of the Order escaped to Cyprus. Theirs is a stirring, romantic story. From Cyprus they took Rhodes, which they held from 1310 to 1523 when the island was captured by Sultan Suleiman the Magnificent. The Knights capitulated and, with all the honours of war, sought refuge in Crete.

Once again they were without a home until 1530, when the Emperor Charles V gave them Malta. There they lived till they were driven out by Napoleon in 1798. Their vast possessions in France had meanwhile been confiscated by the Revolution. The history of this Order now virtually ends. The Grand Priory in the British Realm of the Most Venerable Order of the Hospital of St. John of Jerusalem, founded in the twelfth century, was reconstructed in 1827. In 1888 it was granted a Royal Charter by Queen Victoria, and Edward VII, while Prince of Wales, served as the first Grand Prior. The Order maintains three foundations: the Ophthalmic Hospital in Jerusalem, the St. John Ambulance Association, and the St. John Ambulance Brigade.

Let us return to the St. John's Sisters. After the fall of Jerusalem they settled in the cloister of Sirena, between Saragossa and Lerida in Spain. They then established a number of houses all over the Continent and in 1583 founded a convent at Malta, which was not connected with any hospital. As a nursing order they have long ceased to exist.

The Teutonic Knights began their existence in a field hospital outside the walls of Acre and were approved by Clement III in 1191. For a time they were under the jurisdiction of the Order of St. John, but their Grand Master was always a German. There were also women members of this Order who were engaged in nursing the sick.

The history of the Knights of St. Lazarus is obscure. We read of them nursing lepers in Jerusalem after the establishment of the Christian Kingdom. There is reliable evidence that there were also Sisters of St. Lazarus. When leprosy gradually ceased to be a formidable medical problem, the need for the specific work of this Order diminished, so it was suppressed by Pope Innocent VIII in 1490, and its possessions were handed over to the Order of St. John. The Order of St. Lazarus was revived in the following century, but was soon combined with other Orders. In 1772 we find records of Dames de S. Lazaire at Cambrai in France. The Knights and the Sisters of St. Lazarus were swallowed by the French Revolution.

The subsequent story of military nursing is so episodic that it must be dismissed very briefly but for a few names, incidents, and anecdotes.

In the many wars that punctuated her reign, Isabella the Catholic of Spain (1451–1504) is said to have introduced tented camp hospitals, which employed 'reliable women' to care for the sick. Her grandson Philip II in several of his campaigns enlisted the assistance of the Brothers of St. John of God.

In the sixteenth century bandages were extremely

scarce in the French army, and we are told that the washing of dirty ones was the spare-time duty of four fat prostitutes.

It is interesting to come across records of women serving the wounded single-handed. Around 1653, for example, Elizabeth Alkin nursed wounded sailors, landed after various naval battles, at Harwich and Ipswich—largely at her own expense. Her unselfish work was appreciated, for she was granted a small pension by the government.

Sir John Pringle in his classic *Observations on the Diseases of the Army* (1753) mentions the presence in the military hospitals of 'nurses' as distinct from surgeons' mates and apothecaries.

There was a regular establishment for female nurses in the English expeditionary force sent to aid the Portuguese against Spain in 1762, under command of Lord Loudoun. The first hospital was set up at Lisbon. One of the surgeons was the great John Hunter. The nursing detachment consisted of a matron, who was paid 2s. 6d. a day, 2 head nurses (1s.), and 18 nurses (6d.).

In 1777, in the War of Independence, General Washington ordered women to be sent to 'attend the sick as nurses'.

Usually, however, what little military nursing there was, was done by the wives of serving or pensioned non-commissioned officers. When an army went overseas on active service, local nurses were engaged, if available. The pay of a nurse serving in an English military hospital towards the middle of the eighteenth century was 5s. a week, while nurses employed casually at out-stations received 6d. a day.

'Nurses' or handy-women were employed at the naval hospitals of Plymouth and Haslar during the eighteenth century at a rate of 2s. 6d. a week. Innocent of education or training, they were doubtful characters, for we read of them smuggling liquor into the wards for the patients, conniving at their escape, and robbing the helpless and the dying. In 1854 they were replaced by male old pensioners whose ideas of nursing were, to say the least, crude.

ARMY NURSING SERVICE

It was not until Florence Nightingale went to Scutari in 1854 with her 38 nurses that a proper nursing service was introduced in the British Army. In 1866 we find the first provision made for the posting of nurses to all military general hospitals. An army nursing service was formed in 1881. In the following year, during the Egyptian campaign, nursing sisters were sent overseas to military hospitals at Gibraltar and Malta. In 1889 it was published in Army Orders that sisters were to be employed in all army hospitals with 100 beds or more. The army nursing service was greatly expanded in the South African War of 1899–1902, and in March 1902 the Queen Alexandra's Imperial Military Nursing Service was established, with Queen Alexandra as the first president. In 1914 the service was only 300 strong, but that same year, 2,223 trained nurses enrolled with the reserve, and 1,800 were sent abroad. By 1919 the service and its reserve had grown to more than 10,000.

When the Second World War broke out, the

total peace establishment of the Q.A.I.M.N.S. in all the military hospitals at home and abroad was 624. Immediately the numbers were increased by the mobilization of the Territorial Army Nursing Service, and with the recruitment of its Reserve the members numbered well over 12,000 during the war. On 10th September 1939 the first six army sisters landed in France; 1,300 were evacuated with the B.E.F. from Dunkirk. In 1941 all members of the Service were granted emergency commissions.

In Florence Nightingale's time it was specifically laid down that nurses were to be attached only to the base hospitals in the war area. In the 1939–45 war the Q.A.s sailed with the army to every theatre of war, loyally and heroically sharing its fortunes. In addition to serving in hospitals, sisters were attached to casualty clearing stations, field ambulances, and hospital ships. Some died on the Anzio beaches in the Italian campaign; some were lost in the evacuation of Singapore, and many were missing. At Hong Kong fourteen remained in enemy hands and some of them were murdered.

In 1949, in recognition of its fine record, the Military Nursing Service became a Corps of the Army named Queen Alexandra's Royal Army Nursing Corps, and its officers were granted regular commissions. In the following year nursing rank titles were changed to the equivalent male rank titles, and other ranks were recruited into the Corps. Princess Margaret later became Colonel-in-Chief of the Corps.

The experience in the last war of certain Australian nurses should never be forgotten. On 12th

February 1942, 65 sailed from Singapore. Their ship was bombed and sunk, and eleven were drowned. The survivors landed on Banka Island on the east coast of Sumatra and fell into Japanese hands; 22 were ordered to walk into the sea and, when they were knee-deep in the water, were mercilessly mowed down with a machine gun. One girl was only wounded; regaining consciousness, she found herself lying on the beach among her dead comrades. She crawled into the jungle for safety, but later gave herself up to the enemy to be reunited with the 32 of her friends who now remained of the original detachment of 65. Their story is a sad one; beri-beri, dengue, malaria, typhoid, dysentery, skin diseases, and malnutrition were rife among them, and four died. It was only on 16th September 1945 that all were finally freed and sent to Singapore, where they were admitted to hospital.

ROYAL NAVAL NURSING SERVICE

In 1884–85 six sisters and four head sisters were appointed by the Admiralty to the Royal Naval Hospital at Haslar, under a matron, and assisted by trained sick-berth staff. The service was reorganized in 1902 as the Queen Alexandra's Royal Naval Nursing Service. Its personnel increased from 91 in 1939 to 1,229 during the Second World War. Besides nursing in naval hospitals in ports at home and abroad, members served in Royal Naval hospital ships, in troop ships, and on naval air stations. After the Japanese capitulation in August 1945 some sisters based with the Pacific Fleet sailed in

D

aircraft carriers and other ships engaged in locating and repatriating ex-prisoners of war from widely scattered places in the Pacific Ocean and the China Seas. Since the establishment of the National Health Service in Great Britain the Royal Naval Medical and Nursing Services in overseas naval bases have extended their work to include the families of men stationed abroad. In Malta six Royal Naval sisters provide a home nursing service for the wives and families of naval men.

AIR FORCE NURSING SERVICE

In the 1914–18 War care of the sick of the Royal Flying Corps was the responsibility of the Army Medical Department, and their nursing was in the hands of the Q.A.I.M.N.S. An Air Force Nursing Service was formed in June 1918 as a war-time measure. It was established as a permanent branch of the R.A.F. on 27th January 1921 and in June 1923 was given the title of the Princess Mary's Royal Air Force Nursing Service. Like all the other services it expanded greatly during the Second World War. Sisters served not only where airmen were based, but as the forces advanced, some were flown with emergency equipment to set up mobile hospitals near newly established air fields. Not only are service men trained to make parachute landings, but Royal Air Force sisters may volunteer for this branch of the service.

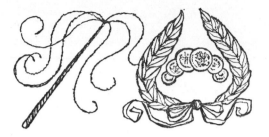

6

Punishments and Rewards

MISDEEDS AND PUNISHMENTS

You can call yourself lucky that you were not a nurse in medieval, or even later, times, for, if you had misbehaved, you might have been made to eat your meals on the floor; you might even have been soundly whipped.

In A.D. 508 St. Césaire d'Arles, founder of a monastery for women, ordained that disobedient nuns be chastised with a rod or a whip. In the same century St. Benedict laid down that 'If a sister that has been several times admonished, will not mend her conduct, let her be excommunicated for a while in proportion; if this kind of correction be useless, let her be chastened by stripes'. In the monasteries and nunneries of early Christianity the whip was the customary implement used liberally and severely for many offences against the rules of those institutions. The 'discipline' was either 'inferior' or 'superior'; the meaning of these terms is obvious.

51

From a statute of the second year of George I of the Irish Parliament, which began on 12th November 1715, we learn that 'ill-conducted nurses' were committed to a house for correction, where they were kept for three months on hard labour, and that they were 'whipt publickly on some market day between the hours of 11 and 12 in the morning through the streets'.[1]

The statutes of the Hôtels-Dieu in Lyons and Paris[2] mention a variety of punishments. The following extracts, translated from the original Latin, may be quoted:

'Therefore whoever is tried and publicly found guilty of disobedience or unchasteness or of retaining his own property without the superior's permission, shall undergo this punishment: for forty days let him be banished from the precincts of the church, and also, being set apart from the common table of the friars, let him sit on the bare ground and eat without any table-cloth, and for those forty days let him fast on bread and water on the fourth and sixth week-days, and only eat meat on Sundays, and do not let him have linen sheets on his bed. . . .

'And what has been said about the discipline of the friars throughout these rules, the same is to be understood of the discipline of the nuns, except that punishment is to be administered to the friars in chapter or in the refectory, but to the nuns by the prioress in the refectory or in the house of the nuns,

[1] Norman Moore: *The History of St. Bartholomew's Hospital*, London, 1918, *ii*, 764 (footnote).

[2] Léon Le Grand: *Statute d'Hôtels-Dieu et de Léproseries*. Recueil de textes du xiie au xvie siècle. Paris, 1901.

or even in the court of the poor, if they have done wrong in public.'

'Once every seven days the nuns as well as the friars shall meet in chapter to hear complaints and administer correction, when at least two shall read and explain the rule of the Order. But if the correction merits corporal punishment, the superior shall punish the friars in the presence of the friars apart from the nuns, and the nuns' superior shall punish the nuns in the presence of the nuns apart from the friars.'

'If any friar has clearly committed fornication outside the house, let him be admonished once, twice and a third time, and if he refuses to abandon and renounce this, let him be driven from the community and, if he repents, let him fast on bread and water on the sixth weekday for seven years unless he is absolved by the direction and favour of the prior, and so too in the case of the nuns.

'If a friar has clearly committed fornication with a nun (God forbid!), let the friar be driven from the house without mercy, whoever he may be; the nun is to be kept in and is to do penance as long as she lives, by being deprived of her habit and by disciplines and fastings in whatever way it shall seem good to her prior and chapter, according to their judgement.'

DIVERSE MISDEEDS

Around 1741 the first nurse to be appointed at the London Hospital 'was reported to have taken money from patients; she was not dismissed, however, as it was not in the rules that she should *not* do so. She promised not to do so again'.

In the following century (1840) a nurse at the Radcliffe Infirmary, Oxford, was given 'notice to quit her office', having, in a quarrel with another nurse at the dinner table, 'caught up the knife with a threatening gesture', but she had previously been guilty of 'many acts of irregularity'. In 1851 a night nurse was dismissed for 'being drunk and other irregular conduct', and in 1871 an assistant nurse, 'having been observed by the House Surgeon permitting a patient to remain with his arm round her waist, was ordered to be severely reprimanded and threatened with instant dismissal in case of any further complaint being made of her conduct'.

A night nurse found 'sleeping on her watch' at St. Mary's Hospital, London, in 1852 was promptly dismissed. In the following year another night nurse, 'having on two occasions been found asleep on her watch, she has been removed from that duty and made an extra assistant nurse'. In 1908 two sisters were censured for allowing dancing in their wards on the evening of Boxing Day!

GENERAL NURSING COUNCILS FOR ENGLAND AND WALES, SCOTLAND AND NORTHERN IRELAND

These statutory bodies, the majority of whose members are registered nurses elected by their colleagues, came into being when the first Nurses Act was passed in 1919. They are entrusted with the approval of hospitals as nurse training schools; they lay down rules regarding the curriculum, length of training, and conduct of examinations; and they maintain registers of qualified nurses. They have the power to erase from the Register the name of any nurse who has been convicted in a civil court and whom they consider to be an unworthy member of the nursing profession. Her name may subsequently be restored on reconsideration.

REWARDS

SALARIES

In the earlier days of hospital nursing in England the hours of work were long and salaries were small.

At St. Bartholomew's Hospital, London, back in 1580 the sisters received 'sixteen pence a wcke and a gowne yerelye for a lyuery', but that same year it was ordered that they have 'two pence more wekely now, toward theyr better releff'.

In 1719 the first matron was appointed at the Westminster Hospital at a salary of £6 a year. Her staff consisted of one nurse (£5 14s.), a maid servant (£4), and a messenger boy (£3). In addition to her administrative duties the matron was day and night nurse. We are told that she received a beer allowance for the patients and the staff amounting to about £3 a month. Apparently, however, the beer was poor, and she spent part of her time watching the nurses lest they slipped in and out with strong beer concealed about their persons. When she resigned because of ill health, she was granted a gratuity of £5.

Talking of beer, at St. Bartholomew's Hospital

the matron sold ale in her house until the practice was forbidden on 22nd January 1559. That it was not suppressed, however, is evident from an order of the Court on 3rd June 1643, 'that there be no tippling in the matron's cellar, and that no beer be kept there'.

At the Westminster Hospital in 1722 Margaret Black was 'entertained as nurse . . . at the rate of eleven shillings a month'.

Guy's Hospital in 1725 had 12 wards with 435 beds. The staff included a matron (£50), 11 sisters (£25), one sister 'belonging to the lunatics' (£25), 8 nurses (£16), and 12 watch-women (£10 8s.). These were higher rates of pay than in other institutions, the intention being to prevent extortion by the staff of money from the patients. In 1738 it was asked: 'Is it necessary to pay a sister £25 per annum and a keeper £35 for looking after 20 lunaticks—surely it is too much!'

In 1894 nurses in training were paid £8 the first year, £12 the second, and £18 the third, and staff nurses £25, £28, and £30, to encourage them to stay on at the hospital after completion of their training.

At the London Hospital the first nurse was appointed about 1741 at a salary of 5s. a week, to live out, and a night nurse at 3s. 6d. The matron was paid £15 a year, plus 6d. a day for each patient, with which to provide food. The salary in 1743 of a resident nurse was £6 per annum, and of 'a watch' £4. In the 1890's probationers received £10 per annum for 80 or more hours a week.

The Radcliffe Infirmary, Oxford, in 1770 paid

its nurses £5 a year, with a gratuity added for good behaviour. In 1847 a nurse aged nearly 75, 'almost past her work', retired on a pension of 4s. a week.

The matron at the General Hospital, Nottingham, in 1783 was given an annual salary of £15, plus 3 guineas for tea and sugar, while the nurses were paid 5 guineas plus a guinea tea and sugar allowance. In 1843 the salary for female nurses was increased to 10 or 12 guineas.

In 1858 it was resolved that the salaries of the sisters at St. Mary's Hospital, London, be raised from £20 to £25 by annual instalments which, however, would only start after they had behaved themselves well for a period of two years. Day nurses were paid a maximum of £18, and night nurses £20 a year. In 1860 the matron's remuneration was £50. After she had held office for six years she asked for an increase, but this was refused. In 1906 a matron was appointed at an annual salary of £150.

The present-day salaries and allowances are laid down in Nurses and Midwives Council Circulars No. 79, 81 and 82. Allowances for student nurses compare favourably with those of students in other professions, and deductions for board, uniforms, and laundry are on a liberal scale.

HOLIDAYS

Information concerning regular holidays for nurses in the early days is difficult to obtain, but it is probable that they were not thought of until late in the nineteenth century. At the Radcliffe Infirmary in 1853 the matron was permitted to grant nurses two or three days during the summer season, according as they could be spared during the painting and cleaning of the wards. In 1874, after their exertions in a fire at the hospital they were allowed three days extra.

At University College Hospital in 1890 the average annual holiday for probationers was two weeks, for staff nurses three weeks, for sisters four weeks.

At Guy's Hospital around 1893 nurses were given two weeks, three weeks, and at the end of the third year and in subsequent years four weeks. Before 1893 the sisters arranged the nurses' half-days; in that year time-tables were drawn up. Sister's week-end was inaugurated in 1898.

The modern regulations for annual leave with pay were framed by the Nurses and Midwives Whitley Council on 1st April 1955.

DECORATIONS

ORDER OF ST. KATHERINE

The Order of St. Katherine was founded by Queen Victoria in 1880 'as a mark of honour for Hospital Nurses, who have particularly distinguished themselves by their good behaviour and attention to duties, and by their aptitude for teaching others'. The recipient of the Order wore a badge on the left arm, consisting of an oval of white surrounded by a border of bright green, and with the letters St. K. in raised gold in the centre; she was given £50 per annum for three years over and above her normal salary, and her hospital received a like sum for her board and lodging. The first three nurses to be decorated with this Order belonged to Westminster Hospital.

ROYAL RED CROSS

The Royal Red Cross was founded on 27th April 1883 by Queen Victoria as a military order for members of the nursing services or other women, British or foreign, recommended for special devotion and competency in nursing with the army in the field, in naval or military hospitals, or hospital ships, etc. On 5th July 1883, 'at Windsor, several of the nurses who attended the sick and wounded during the Egyptian and Zulu campaigns received from the Hands of Her Majesty the decoration of the Royal Red Cross'. (*Lancet*, 1883, *ii*, 85.) The badge is a cross pattée of crimson gilt-edged enamel, having on the arms 'Faith, Hope, Charity' and the date of the award in base with the effigy of the Monarch in relief in gold in the centre for the first class and in frosted silver for the second. The reverse of the centre shows the royal and imperial cipher with crown. There are now two classes, 'members' and 'associates'. Members are trained nurses, but associates need not be.

THE MILITARY MEDAL

This was instituted by royal warrant in 1916 for award to non-commissioned officers and men of the

British Forces for bravery in the field. Women were made eligible by a later warrant. In the Second World War a number of nurses received this decoration for conspicuous devotion to duty during air raids.

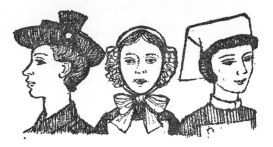

7

The Nurse's Uniform

One of the earliest references in existence to the dress worn by a predecessor of yours in the fourth century A.D. is highly critical: a letter written by St. John Chrysostom, Archbishop of Constantinople, to a woman worker of his, the beautiful, wealthy, and fanatically ascetic Olympia, comments on 'the unspeakable coarseness of thy attire, the shapelessness, the carelessness of thy garments, of thy shoes'.

About that time nursing sisterhoods began to be founded in large numbers. In the beginning their members wore no distinctive dress, and quite as late as the close of the tenth century nuns dressed similarly to the laity. We read of abbesses and nuns of royal birth donning magnificent raiments for state occasions. The religious habits worn by women date from the thirteenth century. If you want a rough idea what these were like, have a look at a nurse working in a modern operating theatre.

Unfortunately, contemporary descriptions of the medieval costume are rather vague. In the ninth and tenth centuries it consisted of a tunic ('kirtle'), put on over the head on top of the only undergarment worn by women. The Saxon name for the latter was 'smock'. The Normans introduced the term 'chemise'. The 'kirtle' was made of linen for the wealthy, and of wool for the poor.

A veil, concealing the hair, was kept on even in bed. Stockings are not specifically mentioned at that time; presumably they were worn, but were carefully concealed under the long tunic. In the eleventh century we have references to stockings of cloth which sometimes extended above the knees.

A century or two later we find mention made of underclothes, the main purpose of which was to protect the outer clothing from the dirty skin! In those days people paid little attention to bodily cleanliness; in fact, the importance of personal hygiene was not appreciated until Beau Brummell's time (1778–1840). It is interesting to observe that in cold weather both men and women kept warm by adding layers to their outer garments, and not by warmer underclothing.

The early history of the petticoat as a separate garment hanging from the waist is not known, but it was well established in England by the sixteenth century. English women began to wear drawers only towards the very end of the eighteenth century, and these became fashionable about 1806. In France, however, ladies habitually wore 'les caleçons' from the middle of the sixteenth century, and in early seventeenth-century Italy, women had 'silke or linnen breeches under their gownes'.

The brassière was first mentioned under that name in 1912; it became known as the 'bra' in 1937.

After this digression let us return to our subject— the nurse's uniform.

The preceding chapters of this book have given us occasional glimpses of how nuns and nurses dressed through the centuries.

In accordance with a papal edict all hospitallers at first wore the black habit with the cowl and the white linen cross of eight points—the signs of the eight beatitudes, 'which thou must ever preserve:

> spiritual joy
> to live without malice
> to weep over thy sins
> to humble thyself to those who injure thee
> to love justice
> to be merciful
> to be sincere and pure of heart
> to suffer persecution'.

At a later period the Knights of St. John wore a white cross—the symbol of purity—on a red ground. The costume of the Sisters of St. John is described in Chapter 5.

With the Beguines, a community of lay nurses founded at Liège in Flanders by the priest Lambert de Bègue about 1170, the adoption of a uniform was optional. At Liège the nurses usually wore grey, and those in other towns blue. At Nîmes in France and at Nivelles in the province of Brabant they used the ordinary attire of the world.

In the early days of the Hôtel-Dieu at Lyons there

was no special uniform. When, however, some nurses appeared in costumes which were a 'cause of scandal', the Rectors in 1526 introduced a uniform white garb. In 1562 this was changed to black with a white linen apron and an unstarched white cap.

The dress of the nursing order of the Hôtel-Dieu in Paris was referred to in Chapter 3. We are told that in the beginning ordinary clothes were worn on duty and that these became more and more gaudy.

At St. Bartholomew's Hospital in London four sisters who formed part of the original body corporate, having joined in the reigns of King John, Henry III, and Edward III, wore the habit of the Augustinian order, and this uniform was to be seen in the hospital for some 400 years. The first matron probably appointed in 1549, wore russet frieze, which four years later she changed to watchett or light blue. This colour, with variations in the depth of the blue, has remained the sisters' uniform to the present day. The sisters, apparently, failed to wear it regularly, for on 15th March 1680, we find an entry in the *Journal* to the effect that the ancient custom of the house was for sisters to wear livery of such coloured cloth or stuff as appointed by the governors, but that it had not been observed of late years, although the sisters were given 22s. 6d. a year to buy it. It was then ordered that all sisters had to wear a livery of such coloured cloth as the governors thought meet, and that any refusing were to be dismissed. Six years later, on 27th March 1686, sisters were directed always to wear their blue cloth liveries.

In 1821 there is an entry recording that a white cloak called a 'night rail' has always been provided for sisters, and this is ordered to be continued. Night rails were worn for going to church, and we read that a sister who died was buried in her night rail. These cloaks were abolished in 1843.

On 21st December 1821 it was resolved that the sisters' dresses be blue, as always before, and the nurses' brown, and these were the colours that greeted the distinguished physician and historian, Sir Norman Moore, when he entered the hospital as a medical student in 1869. The blue colour for the sisters still continues, but the student nurses today wear light grey, and striped uniform after passing their first examination, with a blue belt added after completing all their examinations.

There is an interesting passage in the Treasurer's report of Guy's Hospital for the period 1856–68: whereas formerly the nurses clothed themselves, the provision of 'indoor uniform dress' has been 'attended with improvement in the respectability of their appearance'. Previously the only indication of a uniform had been a round tin medal, inscribed with the name of the ward and the status of the nurse, and hung round the neck over the clothes. Outdoor uniform was then provided until the end of the century, and all nurses had to wear this when leaving and re-entering the hospital gates.

In 1924 provision was made at Guy's for a State-Registered Nurses' uniform and badge, which were protected by law. This was five years after the passing of the Nurses Registration Act, 1919, according to which 'Any person who not being a person duly registered under this Act, . . . takes or uses the name or title of registered nurse, either alone or in combination with any other words or letters, or any name, title, addition, description, uniform, or badge, implying that he is registered under this Act or is recognised by law as a registered nurse; . . . shall be liable on summary conviction to a fine not exceeding, in the case of a first offence, ten pounds, and in the case of a second or any subsequent offence fifty pounds.'

The *British Medical Journal* (1925, *i*, 716 'Medical Notes in Parliament') records: 'The Chartered Association (Protection of Names and Uniforms) Bill, which passed through Committee in the House of Lords on April 6th, is designed to prohibit the wearing by unauthorized persons of the uniforms of nursing and other associations.'

An amusing story is told about The Middlesex Hospital in the 1870's. The 'Lady Probationers' then wore a dress of violet hue, with a small train three inches long, which swept the floor behind them. To prevent these ornamental encumbrances from becoming soiled and frayed, as they quickly did, their owners used to turn up the hems. When the lady superintendent, Godiva Miriam Thorold, discovered this practice, she soon put a stop to it. 'I devised this little train', she told the offender, 'so that, when you lean over a bed to attend to your patient, your ankles will be covered and the students will not be able to see them.'

This chapter may conclude with an annotation 'The attire of nurses' from the *British Medical Journal*, 1883, *ii*, 737. After admitting that nurses' uniforms have improved during the last twenty-five years, the anonymous critic goes on to say:

The Nurse's Uniform

'Persons who are ill usually have time to notice, and usually are so hyper-sensitive as to be fretted by a great many comparatively minor details which do not annoy those who are whole, even when they attract their attention. . . . Why should the colour of the nurses' dress usually be black? That lugubrious tint can neither please the senses of the sick nor awaken happy associations in their minds. Dresses of some bright and pretty patterns would be far preferable to the melancholy garments now affected by many hospital nurses, and especially by some who belong to ecclesiastical sisterhoods. Apart from its colour, there is one cardinal quality of a nurse's dress which is not always to be found: the texture of the garments ought to be so soft that the dress adapts itself noiselessly to the movements of its wearer, and does not keep up that monotonous rustling which is so peculiarly irritating to nervous patients. . . .

'Heels added to boots or shoes give a stumping noise in walking peculiarly their own. A nurse should wear slippers, without heels, and made of a material so soft as never to give a suspicion of a creak.'

In modern times uniforms have been progressively simplified to be more practical and more hygienic. The process of simplification was particularly drastic during the Second World War: frills were discarded, the cap alone being retained as the symbol of the nurse. The distinctive uniforms of many training schools were reluctantly changed, though some still bear a resemblance to those originally worn. Nightingale nurses at St. Thomas's Hospital continue to wear the mauve striped dress chosen by Florence

Nightingale, and the London Hospital nurses still have the full sleeves of the fashionable dress of the 1870's.

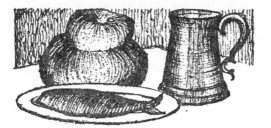

8

Of Bread and Beer

If you had been nursing in some of the London hospitals a century ago, you would have received, in addition to your wages, the sum of eight shillings a week instead of your board. You cooked and ate your meals in the ward kitchen. 'If the sister happened to be partial to red-herrings for breakfast, onion-stew for dinner, or toasted cheese for supper, the consequent state of the ward may be imagined.'[1]

The idea of giving board wages to the nursing staff is a very old one. In 1586, for example, the cook (promoted from a sister!) at St. Bartholomew's Hospital received an additional £4 a year for her diet, and in 1649 we find it recorded: 'granted upon the petition of the fifteen sisters . . . for their future encouragement . . . that their board wages of three shillings per week be increased to three shillings and sixpence a week'. After 8th January 1839, nurses at this hospital were given dinner every day instead of

[1] *British Medical Journal*, 1874, *i*, 285.

Sundays only. In 1870 all the sisters were paid 1s. 6d.
a week more, when certain quantities of meat, bread,
and potatoes, which they used to receive, were abolished.

At the London Hospital in 1742 it was 'agreed
that the matron and the messenger be allowed their
diet from this day at the rate of 2d. loaf per day, and
double the quantity of cheese or butter allowed to
patients'.

According to *The Lancet* Sanitary Commission
Report on Night-Nursing in the London Hospitals
(*Lancet*, 1871, *ii*, 784), at 'The London' the night-
nurses in those days were allowed money instead of
rations and were permitted to do a little cooking in
the lobbies attached to the wards. 'One ward was
rather strongly pervaded with the odour of a raw
onion, which the night-nurse was eating as a relish
with her tea.'

Three years later, the *British Medical Journal*
(1874, *i*, 286) informs us that 'The old plan of giving
board wages to the nurse is now nearly extinct . . . it
led to most injudicious attempts at economy on the
part of the nurses, to peculations from the patients'
diets, and was the cause of frequent quarrels. It still
lingers in a modified form at St. Bartholomew's; the
sisters there have still to provide the greater part of
their food, while the nurses receive uncooked rations
of meat, flour, vegetables, etc.' We are also told that
at Guy's the nurses received three dresses, but that
'butter is an extra'.

Talking of Guy's, the Treasurer's Report 1856–
68 states that formerly, apart from an allowance of
bread and beer, the nurses boarded themselves, but

that the provision of full board 'has been attended with improvement in the health of the nurses'. In 1894 the diet was 'improved' by the addition of pudding every day for dinner and by the more frequent supply of cold meat for supper. Chairs were also substituted for the old benches in the dining hall.

Around 1770 the nurses at the Radcliffe Infirmary in Oxford had breakfast in their own rooms or with the patients. At 2 p.m. they went to the servants' hall for dinner which they ate 'in company with the others in the House, including those hired by the day'; they then returned to the wards, taking back a plate of meat and vegetables to serve as their supper. Until about 1880 they were allowed one pint of beer a day, but as a 'fortification against illness' the doctor in charge of a particularly trying case was empowered to order the nurse on duty 'that ration of whatever quality of beer or porter he may judge to be expedient to be issued to such nurse'.

The daily supply of beer at the General Hospital, Nottingham, was more generous than at the Radcliffe, for each inmate, whether male or female, patient or member of the staff, was allowed $2\frac{1}{2}$ pints. In 1839 the nurses were given $\frac{1}{2}$ pint at lunch, 1 pint at dinner, and 1 pint at supper. Tea was not provided, but the matron and the nurses received tea money.

At the Bristol Royal Infirmary in 1866, a room which had formerly served as a museum and subsequently as a convalescent ward for men, was furnished with a long table and chairs and converted into a nurses' dining-room. Each nurse was provided by the housekeeper with $\frac{1}{2}$ lb. of butter a week; this she kept in her ward and brought with her to all meals.

At breakfast she received a 12-oz. loaf of bread which had to last for the day and of which she took what she required into the ward for her tea. For this repast, which could be had whenever it was found convenient, each nurse was allowed 3 oz. of tea and ½ lb. of loaf sugar a fortnight. In 1890 the tea allowance was increased to 4 oz. a week. In 1893 fish and bacon were served for breakfast, in addition to eggs, and two years later butter in small pats was placed on the table, with no restriction as to the amount used. Dinner in 1866 consisted of meat and potatoes every day, with soup twice a week, and a second vegetable or milk pudding two or three times weekly. For supper there was cold meat, bread and cheese, and ½ pint of beer. It is significant to find no mention made of fresh fruit.

An extract from *Eastern Hospitals and English Nurses* by a Lady Volunteer (1856) sheds interesting light on the nurse's diet, both solid and liquid, in the Crimean war:

'We suffered greatly for want of proper food. Our diet consisted of the coarse sour bread of the country, tea without milk, butter so rancid we could not touch it, and very bad meat and porter; and at night a glass of wine or brandy.'

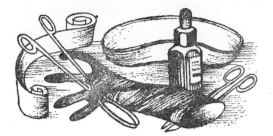

9

The Nurse's Daily Tools

Apart from the vast—and to the student nurse, bewildering—array of surgical instruments which she has to handle when on duty in the operating theatre, the nurse uses several professional tools which are part of her everyday life in the wards, in 'casualty', and in 'out-patients'. Some of these have curious and even romantic histories.

RUBBER GLOVES

The tale of the introduction of rubber gloves into surgery is of particular interest to nurses. Rubber gloves are usually regarded as one of the measures adopted by the surgeon to prevent infection of the patient on whom he is operating. They were, however, first used for a more sentimental reason. It is the old story of 'Cherchez la femme'. The traditional 'hero' of this romance is the American surgeon William Stewart Halsted of Johns Hopkins Hospital, Baltimore—a pioneer who established a school of surgery founded on the results of scientific experiment. There is also a 'heroine', for Halsted introduced gloves not to protect the patient on the operating table from the surgeon's hands, but to protect the sensitive hands of his theatre nurse from the strong antiseptic solutions then in fashion. The nurse was Caroline Hampton, a shy, tall, dark-eyed, efficient girl who had been appointed head nurse in Halsted's operating room at the hospital in 1889 shortly after she had graduated from the New York Hospital. In those days the ritual of 'scrubbing up' was both complicated and strenuous: first the hands and arms were vigorously scrubbed for five to ten minutes with green soap and water, using a stiff brush; next they were dipped in a saturated aqueous solution of potassium permanganate, which coloured them a chocolate brown; then they were soaked in oxalic acid solution which, by oxidizing the permanganate, restored the normal colour of the skin; finally, they were held for five minutes in a basin filled with a 1 in 1,000 bichloride of mercury solution. All this played havoc with Nurse Hampton's hands, causing a severe dermatitis which made her life so miserable that she complained to her 'Chief'. Other people also were apparently affected in the same way, but they did not voice their grievances.

Gallant Halsted considered his nurse's trouble proof of her aristocratic blood, for she came of an old southern family. At first nothing that he could suggest had the slightest effect. But one day—and by then he had been attracted to her in his curiously formal and undemonstrative way—the idea occurred to him of having rubber gloves made for her, as an experiment. From plaster casts of her hands, which he himself took to New York, the Goodyear Rubber Company supplied two pairs of loose-fitting rubber gauntlet gloves. These served their purpose so well —they also had the advantage that they could be boiled—that in course of time more gloves were ordered, and then a young assistant, whose duty it was to place the surgical instruments in metal trays filled with carbolic acid, took to wearing them. Halsted himself began using thin, close-fitting gloves only some five years later, in 1896, and then but occasionally, for he believed that they interfered with his sensitivity of touch. Sometimes in the middle of an operation he would deliberately remove a glove when undertaking a particularly delicate palpation or exploration.

The general adoption of gloves by surgeons aroused considerable controversy, of which a letter published in the *Medical Record, New York* (1898, 53, 608) may be quoted as an eloquent witness, though hardly as a literary masterpiece. 'Gloves for employment in aseptic surgical work', wrote Robert Tuttle Morris, professor of surgery in the New York Post-Graduate Medical College, 'have been recently advocated on theoretical grounds by so many prominent surgeons that many of the younger men feel in duty bound to use such gloves in order to be up-to-date. To all such younger men who have misgivings prompted by natural sense, I wish to state that one surgeon at least can be depended upon to fortify them by his example in refusing to adopt anything that will injure the surgeon's

most precious possession—the sense of touch. . . .
Surgeons who were doing first-class work three
years ago seem to me to be doing second- or third-
rate work now on account of the interference made
by their gloves. The greatest danger to be feared is
that the younger generation of surgeons may fail
to develop the sense of touch to the highest degree,
and we shall have much second-rate work done,
particularly in abdominal surgery. . . . To the younger
generation of surgeons, I say, fight with your might
against the idea of using a means that will damage
your most precious possession—the sense of touch.
Put aside the temptation to be up-to-date theoretic-
ally, at the cost of adopting a destructive agent in
your work.'

That was nearly sixty years ago. Since then young
surgeons the world over have been brought up with
gloves, and their sense of touch has from the very
beginning developed through gloved hands.

But we must return to Halsted and Caroline
Hampton. The girl whose delicate hands inspired
this surgical advance did not remain a theatre nurse
for long. She and Halsted were married in June
1890 and lived together what has been described as
'a life of aristocratic chill'. The two had much in
common: both were eccentric and difficult, and few
other people were at ease with them. To the end of
his days Halsted never ceased to express surprise
that Caroline should have married a man so unworthy
of her as himself; which, as one of his colleagues at
Johns Hopkins remarked, was after all the correct
attitude for a husband to adopt.

Histories of medicine are full of inaccuracies, and

mistakes are copied from one book to another. It is often stated that cotton or silk gloves preceded rubber ones, but this is not true. In 1896 Johann von Mikulicz-Radecki, professor of surgery in the University of Breslau, who is internationally known for his two-stage method of resecting a cancer of the large intestine and for 'Mikulicz's disease' (symmetrical inflammation of the lacrimal and salivary glands), began to use fine-thread gloves of the cheapest sort, which could be sterilized by steam. About the same time the Leipzig surgeon Georg Clemens Perthes started wearing silk gloves with a rubber covering. By then rubber gloves had already been in experimental use for at least five years.

To complete the story, rubber gloves in obstetrics were first used in 1898 by Albert Döderlein of Tübingen, but it is interesting to recall that as early as 1758 Johann Georg Walbaum of Lübeck wore gloves made of sheep's caecum when performing a version.

THE THERMOMETER

No task is performed in the wards more regularly and more universally than the taking of temperatures. The clinical thermometer is the nurse's most familiar tool—easy to use and easy to break. In its present form it is less than a hundred years old. What did its precursors look like?

The marked changes in temperature that occur in the course of many diseases could hardly have escaped the notice of the early physicians, but the story of medical thermometry really begins in the seventeenth century. About 1625 an Italian physician Santorio Santorio, or Sanctorius, of Padua (for generations Padua was the nursery of learning) constructed, and advocated the use of, a mouth thermometer for diagnosing disease. He also correlated variations in temperature with variations in weight and first described 'insensible perspiration', thus founding the physiology of metabolism.

The next figure of importance, a century later, is the illustrious Dutch doctor Hermann Boerhaave, who first expounded the principles of medical thermometry. His pupil Gerard van Swieten of Vienna advised that the heat of fever be recorded by thermometers, as the sensitivity of the physician's hand was far from trustworthy, and he himself used the mercurial thermometer introduced by G. D. Fahrenheit, for taking temperatures in the mouth and under the arm. As Victor Robinson graphically put it, the Old Vienna School grew up under van Swieten with a thermometer in its mouth.

During the eighteenth century a number of Englishmen made valuable experimental observations on body and environmental temperatures. One of these was the great John Hunter whose bust you can see over the entrance to St. George's Hospital Medical School at Hyde Park Corner.

The next important step was made by James Currie of Liverpool, author of *Medical Reports, on the Effects of Water, Cold and Warm, as a Remedy in Fever and Febrile Diseases* (1797)—a medical classic based on personally observed cases and on the older literature. He was one of the first to direct attention to the value of repeated thermometric

records in fever. In his day there was no self-register-
ing thermometer, and the temperature had to be
read with the instrument *in situ*. Currie modified the
thermometer used by John Hunter—a stout glass
stem with a small bulb—by bending it at an angle
and enabling him to read it in the axilla or under the
tongue, while standing behind the patient. No one
took any notice of his pioneer work. It was a treatise
published in 1868 by Carl Wunderlich of Württem-
berg that laid the foundation of modern clinical
thermometry. Thermometry now became a recognized part of diagnosis. Of Wunderlich it has been
well said that he found fever a disease and left it a
symptom.

Clinical thermometers were a novelty in the wards
of English hospitals around 1866. And what a
novelty they were! Fearsome instruments, ten inches
long and carried under the arm like a gun. They
took five minutes to register the axillary temperature.

The short clinical thermometer which we use today was introduced in 1867 by Thomas Clifford
Allbutt of Leeds. His original instrument measured
six inches and was carried in a wooden stethoscope.
Later it was shortened to four, and then to three
inches, and the time required to obtain a reading
was gradually reduced to thirty seconds.

Who can tell what changes this familiar tool will
undergo in the years to come? Recently an electrical
thermometer has been designed with a metallic
probe serving as a heat conductor and giving an
accurate reading time of thirteen seconds. Similar in
size and shape to the ordinary mercury thermometer,
but connected by means of a flex to an indicating

instrument, it is constructed of platinum, silver, and platinum-iridium, the cost of which makes it impractical for routine use.[1]

HIGGINSON'S SYRINGE

All nurses have heard of Higginson's syringe, but few realize that it has been in use for 100 years.

The enema has a long history, so long that its beginnings are lost in the mists of antiquity. It was popular with the ancients—Egyptians, Sumerians, Chinese, Greeks, and Romans. From time to time the old fallacy is revived that the Egyptians borrowed the idea of the enema from the ibis—a fallacy repeated by the famous Dutch physician Regnier de Graaf, who wrote in his classic *Tractatus de Clysteribus* (1668): 'We know there is in Egypt a bird called the Ibis, not unlike a stork, which first showed us the use of the clyster. This creature, conscious of being heavy with a mass of noxious humours, fills its beak with sea water and washes out that part which is the natural outlet for the over-loaded belly, making it wholesome.'[2] What really happens, however, is that the ibis, when preening its feathers, dips its long beak into water and then collects oil from glands near the anus.

Enemas were given by the Greeks and Romans by means of metal syringes without valves. Manual pressure on a collapsible bag was another method

[1] *Nursing Mirror*, 17th August, 1956, *103*, 1,432.
[2] This passage is taken from William Brockbank and O. R. Corbett: 'De Graaf's "Tractatus de Clysteribus",' *Journal of the History of Medicine*. 1954, *9*, 178.

used during the Renaissance, and liquid from receptacles of pottery, glass, or metal was also introduced by atmospheric pressure at that time. In the middle of the seventeenth century two types of enema syringe were commonly employed: an ox-bladder fastened to a pipe and holding 'one wine pint' of fluid, and a syringe made of pewter. Both had obvious disadvantages: the former was difficult to handle and had a tendency to burst at the wrong moment; the second could be painful and dangerous.

According to the French army surgeon Ambroïse Paré, in 1580 the enema syringe was in such common use in every country that physicians thought it more befitting to their dignity not to sully their hands with it. It had become an instrument most used by surgeons who in those days were people of much inferior status. For the benefit of patients who were too modest to expose their buttocks Paré invented an instrument 'with which one may give a clyster to himself by putting the pipe into the fundament'.

The clyster reached the height of its popularity in the reign of Louis XIV of France (1638–1715), who is believed to have had over 2,000 enemas in his life.

The syringe invented in the 1850's by Higginson (known on the continent as the 'English syringe'), was provided with valves which were thought to make injection under pressure a simple and safe procedure, because the amount of fluid entering the rectum could be controlled. Alfred Higginson, M.R.C.S., L.S.A., L.M. (1808–84), was on the surgical staff of the Liverpool Southern Hospital (now the Royal Southern Hospital) from 1857–67. This dexterous, careful, and ingenious surgeon also invented a stomach pump, an ether inhaler, and a valved syringe for vein-to-vein blood transfusion. With his long beard, bushy eyebrows, and piercing eyes he looked like Charles Darwin. His syringe is no longer used, as there is a very real danger of injuring the rectum. It has been replaced by a simple funnel and soft rubber catheter.

THE HYPODERMIC SYRINGE

Do not ask, 'Who invented the hypodermic syringe?', for you will not get a satisfactory answer. The hypodermic syringe which doctors and nurses use today cannot properly be said to have been invented by one man. Its story is interesting, but not easy to unravel.

The importance of hypodermic medication is well known to all experienced nurses. For years it has been the means by which a patient with a severe injury or in the terminal stages of an inoperable cancer, for example, has found merciful relief from his pain. It enables drugs to be given for rapid action with far greater control than do other methods. More recently it has played its part in the miracles wrought every day in hospital wards since the advent of chemotherapy. Hypodermic insulin injections allow the diabetic to lead a near-normal life, and hypodermic premedication allays the fears of the nervous patient about to undergo an operation.

It is intriguing to speculate whether the bites of poisonous snakes and insects first suggested the introduction of medicaments into the human body through a skin puncture. Of all the routes used for administering drugs—the mouth, by swallowing or inhalation, the rectum, the urethra, the veins, or subcutaneous tissue—the hypodermic route was the last to be adopted, just over a century ago.

Intravenous injections were first suggested in 1656 to Robert Boyle by Christopher Wren, the architect of St. Paul's Cathedral. One of the earliest recorded therapeutic hypodermic injections was given in 1844 by Francis Rynd of the Meath Hospital, Dublin, who used acetate of morphine to relieve a woman of trigeminal neuralgia. But it was only in 1861 that he published details of his instrument—a simple trocar and cannula. By that time the hypodermic syringe was well established. Unaware of Rynd's work, Alexander Wood of Edinburgh, in November 1853, cured an elderly spinster suffering from 'cervico-brachial neuralgia' by injecting a solution of muriate of morphine. Ferguson of Giltspur Street, London, made him a small syringe which was the first to be fitted with a hollow needle. It was while using it to inject an acid solution of perchloride of iron for the removal of a naevus, that the possible usefulness of this instrument for administering a narcotic occurred to him. Wood had no other idea than to obtain a local effect of the drug on the nerves close to the site of the injection. He was aware that this method must also produce some general effect, but seems to have overlooked the clinical importance of the fact. His classic 'New Method of Treating Neuralgia' was published in 1855.

The first person to recognize that in order to relieve pain there is no need to inject a drug subcutaneously in the region where the pain is, but that it may be injected anywhere in the body, was Charles Hunter, house-surgeon at St. George's Hospital, London. This was only three years after the publication of Wood's book, and there followed a bitter, and at times undignified, controversy between the two, from which Hunter emerged the winner.

Where does Charles Gabriel Pravaz of Lyons (1791–1853) come into the story? The curiously persistent legend that he invented hypodermic medication has been exploded by N. Howard-Jones,[1] who showed that Pravaz used a syringe of a type already in common use and was concerned solely with the injection of blood coagulants for the cure of aneurysm.

Very few discoveries in medicine can justly be attributed to one man alone. Most of them have been made by men who were clever enough to see new possibilities in ideas or in materials already in existence. Wood's claim to remembrance is his adoption of the subcutaneous route for administering drugs. Charles Hunter grasped the idea of obtaining general effects by injection, and he introduced the term 'hypodermic'.

URINE TESTING

Examination of the urine as an aid to diagnosis dates from very early times. The Jewish physician and philosopher Isaac Israeli of Tunisia, usually known as Isaac Judaeus (A.D. *c*. 845–*c*. 940), wrote one of the first books on uroscopy, but for centuries

[1] *Journal of the History of Medicine*, 1947, 2, 201–49.

thereafter inspection of the urine remained a completely unscientific and highly speculative procedure. The Arabian physicians pretended to tell the sex of the unborn child by looking at the mother's urine. 'Water-casting' as it was called, is a favourite theme in many famous Dutch paintings of the seventeenth century. Jan Steen, for example, has left nine pictures in which he depicts a physician examining the urine of a girl suffering from the so-called *mal d'amour* or the chlorosis of lovesick maidens. There is a charming picture by Gerard Dou in Buckingham Palace, showing a handsome young doctor, magnificently dressed in furs, earnestly gazing at a urine-flask and at the same time feeling the pulse of a pretty girl, whose interest in the man is obviously far greater than her confidence in his professional ability.

Mal d'amour and green-sickness were old names for what is now recognized as an iron-deficiency anaemia (chlorosis) developing in girls at the age of puberty. The term 'chlorosis', derived from the Greek for 'green', was applied to the condition because of the greenish pallor which was one of its chief characteristics. The first clear description is attributed to Johann Lange of Silesia (*De morbo virgineo*, 1554). There are many references in literature to pale, green-sick, lovelorn, and feverish maidens, and love was often blamed for their low spirits, and lack of vitality. Chlorosis has now almost entirely disappeared, largely because girls today lead far healthier lives than did those of the sixteenth century.

The Turin Codex of the *El Hawi* of Rhazes contains a magnificent miniature which shows one of the masters of the medical school of Salerno inspecting urine in a glass, while the patient stands by holding the urine basket in which he has brought the specimen. These baskets, made of osier and fitted with a lid and handle, were in common use when the practice of uroscopy was in vogue.

It is interesting to reflect that modern pregnancy tests had their medieval counterpart when 'water-casting' was employed in the diagnosis of chastity.

One of the first to adopt more scientific methods was Lorenzo Bellini of Florence (1643–1704), who insisted on chemical analysis of the urine in disease. Before him the Belgian physician-chemist Jean Baptiste van Helmont (1577–1644) had introduced gravimetric analysis of urine: he made a practice of weighing twenty-four hour specimens,[1] but was unable to draw any scientific deductions from his figures.

The man who did more than any one to stimulate interest in the chemistry of the urine was Johann Florian Heller of Vienna (1813–71). He invented the ureometer for estimating specific gravity, devised the ring test for albumen known by his name, and was the first to note the retention of chlorides in the urine of patients with pneumonia. His book on urinary concretions was long a classic. A contemporary of Heller's, Hermann von Fehling, described his test for the presence of sugar in the urine in 1848. Some of the other routine tests which we use today

[1] The 24-hour specimen is a patient's urinary output for a whole day and night. The bladder is emptied at the beginning of the period, but this specimen is discarded. All subsequent specimens are collected in a large Winchester quart bottle.

are comparatively recent. Benedict's test for sugar was introduced in 1907 by the American biochemist Stanley Rossiter Benedict, and a year later A. C. H. Rothera of Melbourne devised his test for acetone bodies.

The days are past when the doctor pinned his faith on visual inspection of the urine and when Sir Thomas Elyot could write in *The Castell of Helth* (1534): 'The most common judgement in sickness is by urines.' Urine, however, still plays an important role in diagnosis, and with ever-improving techniques its examination yields information of a nature unsuspected by the ancients.

In recent years urinalysis has been considerably simplified for nurse, doctor, and patient by the development of six standardized tests: Clinitest, Clinistix, Acetest, Albustix, Occultest, Ictotest (Ames Company (London) Ltd.).

DRESSINGS

Much of the nurse's time in the wards and in the out-patients department was taken up with dressings, and in the course of her training she had ample opportunities of observing the effects of various types on the healing of wounds.

Surgical dressings have a long and fascinating history. When primitive man cut himself or was injured by an enemy, human or animal, he dressed his wound with leaves or grass. The ancient Egyptians used fresh meat and honey. In many parts of the world healing virtues were attributed to cow-dung. The School of Hippocrates in Greece advocated simple cleanliness to prevent wounds from suppurating. This teaching, however, was rapidly forgotten until that remarkable man, Theodoric of Lucca, medical practitioner and bishop of Cervia in Italy, in the thirteenth century A.D. recommended simple substances like wine to speed the process of healing. At that time surgeons were under the spell of the doctrine of 'laudable pus', as it was called, according to which every wound, while healing, normally produced pus. Theodoric's teaching also fell on deaf ears, and not until 700 years later did Lord Lister finally revolutionize surgery by introducing the antiseptic system, whose logical outcome was aseptic surgery. When Lister was a medical student, the superstition of 'laudable pus' was still very much alive, and he had to fight the same battle that Theodoric of old had fought.

GAMGEE TISSUE

Until some seventy-five years ago the poultice was a popular surgical dressing. It had to be renewed daily, for it was non-absorbent, the wound was rapidly infiltrated by discharge, and the whole thing became a damp, warm, sodden mass. It was a clinical lecture delivered to the medical students at Birmingham on February 18th, 1880 that dethroned the poultice from general favour and introduced a novel, dry, absorbent, infrequently renewed dressing which has since become a household word. Joseph Sampson Gamgee qualified, like his father, as a veterinary surgeon before studying medicine at University College, London. In 1855 he was appointed surgeon to the British Italian Legion and took charge of the hospital at Malta in the Crimean War. He was elected to the surgical staff of the Queen's Hospital, Birmingham, in 1857, and he is said to have been one of the first, if not the first, in that city to wash his hands before dressing a wound or operating as well as after. A brilliant linguist, he could read a scientific paper before a French, German, Spanish, or Italian society without the members realizing that he was a foreigner.

The idea of a dry absorbent dressing occurred to Gamgee while he was reading the chapter on muslin and cotton wool in the 'racy and most instructive essays' on 'Simplified Surgery' published at Brussels in 1842 by Matthias Mayor of Lausanne. This idea he was able to translate into reality when a firm of cotton-wool makers brought to his notice a method of making cotton wool and gauze absorbent by extracting the grease. 'Gamgee Tissue', as it came to be called, consists of a layer of absorbent cotton wool between two layers of absorbent gauze. It possesses the virtues of compression and absorption. You will love Gamgee's description:[1]

'There must be no squeezing like that of an old college friend's hand, when seen after a long absence. The soothing surgical pressure is like that which you interchange with the hand of a lady, when the pleasure of meeting her is tempered by a respectful regard. Your hand adapts itself to hers, and gently presses it wherever it can touch it, but nowhere squeezes it for fear of offending. Such pressure when

[1] *On the Treatment of Wounds and Fractures: Clinical Lectures.* 2nd ed. London, 1883, p. 186.

employed by the surgeon in the treatment of injuries, always soothes and heals.'

SCOTT'S DRESSING

Scott's (a still earlier) dressing is still used occasionally in out-patient departments. Composed of equal parts of soft soap and camphorated mercurial ointment, its employment in chronic joint disease was first advocated in 1828 by John Scott in his book *Surgical Observations on Chronic Inflammations and Diseases of Joints*. His method was to wash the affected limb with hot water and soft soap, to rub it with camphorated spirits of wine, and to cover it with lint on which camphorated mercurial ointment had been thickly spread. An important part of the treatment was the careful application of firm bandages. In an age when bandaging was practised assiduously by the doctor, Scott was reputed the best bandager in London. The son of a general practitioner, he was born at Bromley, Kent, in 1799. He was surgeon to the London Hospital from 1831 to 1845, and surgeon to Moorfields Eye Hospital from 1826 until his death in 1846.

UNNA'S PASTE

Ulcerated legs and their treatment are an ever-present problem, and in all general hospitals large numbers of patients with this trouble are seen in the wards and in the out-patients. At one time a popular remedy was Unna's paste, the formula for which is gelatin 3 parts, zinc oxide 3 parts, glycerin 5 parts, water 9 parts. It is valuable as a soothing protectant which reduces the risk of secondary infection and, incorporated with bandages, provides a good support in varicose ulcers. Paul Gerson Unna (1850–1929), its inventor, gave up general practice to specialize in dermatology. He built a hospital for diseases of the skin in Hamburg, where students and medical practitioners from all over the world came for instruction. In 1919 the University of Hamburg created a chair of dermatology for him.

ANTISEPTICS

With the establishment of the germ theory of disease it became part of nursing practice to apply various antiseptics to wounds. *A Text-Book of Nursing* by C. S. Weeks-Shaw (Edited by W. J. Radford, 3rd impression, London, 1869) mentions in order of merit bichloride of mercury (corrosive sublimate), and carbolic acid, and the following 'also rans' 'of more or less efficiency': salicylic acid, boric acid, biniodide of mercury, creolin, iodine, iodoform, thymol, and the chlorides of lime, soda, and zinc. It draws attention to the danger of toxic symptoms arising from the absorption of carbolic acid and corrosive sublimate through wound dressings.

Progress in bacteriology and the development of a more scientific approach to the problem of wound treatment led to a search for better antiseptics. As with so many advances in medicine and surgery, the exigencies of war stimulated much fruitful research on this question. During the 1914–18 war surgeons had to treat many patients with seriously contaminated wounds, particularly those with gas-gangrene infection. Apart from the loss of life resulting from such infections, many limbs had to be amputated which might have been saved had proper facilities been available for the control of sepsis. One of the men who set himself the task of finding a cheap, but efficient antiseptic first-aid dressing was James Lorrain Smith, professor of pathology at the University of Edinburgh. He succeeded in preparing a powder—a mixture of boric acid and chlorinated lime—that could be sprinkled on a wound immediately, when the moisture would liberate the active antiseptic agent, chlorine. This powder he called 'Eupad'—a contraction for *E*dinburgh *U*niversity *Pa*thological *D*epartment. Later the powder was supplemented by the solution which was christened 'Eusol'—a contraction for *E*dinburgh *U*niversity *Sol*ution.

Eusol has lost some of its popularity because of its irritant properties to skin and epithelium.

The Second World War saw the introduction of a novel local antiseptic which was first successfully tried out on the Normandy Beaches in 1944— nitrofurazone.

DRESSINGS TODAY

Modern dressings have become considerably simplified. Dry gauze dressings are extensively used today, for it is realized that moist dressings tend to encourage the growth of germs. In the first-aid treatment of burns, for example, dry dressings are preferred to those wrung out in normal saline or sodium bicarbonate solution. Clean operation wounds require aseptic dressings of sterile gauze. *Tulle gras* is convenient for dressing minor burns of the face and hands. Plastic spray paints are popular: they make conventional bandages unnecessary; being transparent, they allow the wound to be observed; elimination of frequent dressings saves time and wound contamination.

Treatment of ulcers has been enormously simplified by the introduction of Elastoplast bandages, Viscopaste, Coltapaste, Ichthopaste, etc., in place of the somewhat messy Unna's paste.

When it is necessary to keep a dressing moist, it may be covered with jaconet, which in turn is covered with wool. Cellophane, often used in place of jaconet, can be sterilized in the autoclave and discarded when soiled.

Injuries to fingers and toes are among the most common forms of accidents. Dressing these has always been difficult, even experts finding the task of bandaging a finger without interfering with its use (to say nothing of its neighbours) something of a problem. The introduction of Tubegauz, which with the aid of a bivalve applicator can be fitted snugly and neatly over the injured finger, has proved a real boon to surgeon, nurse, and patient.

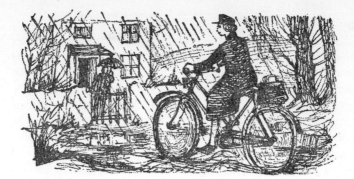

10

The Story of District Nursing

The origins of District or Visiting Nursing must be looked for in the early chronicles of Christianity. From the very beginning visiting the sick was regarded as a religious duty which until the last century, was carried out by the religious orders.

A Roman Catholic Order of Sisters of Mercy was founded in 1831 by Catherine McAuley, who in 1828 had already formed a secular body at Dublin. Her Sisters nursed the Dublin poor during the terrible cholera epidemic in 1832, and in 1847 did heroic work when Liverpool was stricken by typhus.

The first organized district nursing in England began in 1840 with the English Protestant Sisters of Charity—subsequently called 'Nursing Sisters'—though the foundation came into being through the labours of a Quaker lady, Elizabeth Fry. The nurses, who were supplied with uniforms and lived in a Home in Devonshire Square, Bishopsgate, took no vows, but visited the sick poor under the direction of the clergy.

In 1845 the famous tractarian leader Edward Bouverie Pusey established the Park Village Community in Regent's Park. The nurses of the community received no special training, and much religious ritual was bound up with their daily routine. The Sisters of Mercy, founded by Priscilla Sellon at Devonport three years later, likewise had no regular training at first. This movement spread to Bethnal Green and to Pimlico, and later, amalgamated with Pusey's community.

In 1847 the eminent London ophthalmologist William Bowman (afterwards Sir William Bowman, Bt.) emphasized the need for a training institute for nurses, and in the following year the community of St. John's House came into existence at 36 Fitzroy Square, in the district of St. John the Evangelist, St. Pancras, from which it took its name. Later the House moved to Norfolk Street, Strand, and in 1907 to Queen Square, Bloomsbury. In 1919 the Nursing Sisters of St. John were taken over by St. Thomas's Hospital as a private nursing organization.

The year 1859 is a memorable one in the history of district nursing, for in that year William Rathbone, a prosperous Liverpool merchant and philanthropist, engaged Mary Robinson, the nurse who had attended his first wife in her last illness, on a trial period of three months to visit poor patients in their own homes in the Liverpool slums. When after much discouragement and many rebuffs her work began to bear fruit, Rathbone tried to recruit other suitable nurses, but found that none were available. He then consulted with the Royal Infirmary Committee and undertook to build at his own expense a training school and home for nurses. Its objects were to train nurses for work in the Infirmary and for visiting the sick poor in their own homes, and also well-to-do private patients. The Liverpool Training School and Home for Nurses in Ashton Street was in operation by May 1st, 1863.

In 1866 Liverpool was divided into eighteen 'districts', and a nurse was allotted to each district— hence the name 'district nursing'. Ladies resident in the city superintended the work of the nurses, paid for their lodgings, and provided medical comforts and food for the sick who were too poor to supply their own needs. In 1876 a matron was placed in charge of each group of nurses, and the groups were concentrated in district homes. In 1898 the district nursing activities of the Training School were transferred to the Liverpool Queen Victoria District Nursing Association which was so-named because the money collected in the city on the occasion of the Queen's Jubilee in 1887 was used to develop district nursing.

The first association to give nurses trained in hospital an exclusive district nursing training was the Metropolitan and National Nursing Association, founded in 1874 by William Rathbone in accordance with Florence Nightingale's *Suggestions for Improving the Nursing Service for the Sick Poor*. Two years later Florence Lees was appointed the first superintendent of the Home at 23 Bloomsbury Square.

Associations similar to the Liverpool body were established at Manchester and at Salford in 1864, and at Leicester in 1867.

The East London Nursing Society was organized in 1868, and in the same year Mrs. Ranyard founded the Ranyard Mission, a nursing branch of the London Bible Women and Nurses' Mission.

Queen Victoria in 1887 devoted £70,000 of the 'Women's Jubilee Gift' to furthering the 'nursing the sick poor in their own homes by means of trained nurses', and, largely through the efforts of Miss Nightingale and of the great surgeon Sir James Paget, who were convinced of the importance of training nurses for district work, the Queen Victoria Jubilee Institute for Nurses was founded. In 1889 it was granted a Royal Charter, adopted the Metropolitan and National Nursing Association as the nucleus in London, and subsequently became affiliated with the Liverpool and other associations. At the Diamond Jubilee in 1897, and on the occasion of the Queen's death in 1901, further sums were given to promote district nursing throughout the British Isles. The greater part of the sum raised as a national memorial to Queen Alexandra also was devoted to this cause.

When Queen Mary became Patron in 1925, the Institute was renamed the Queen's Institute of District Nursing, and in 1932 it was provided by the National Birthday Trust with new quarters at 57 Lower Belgrave Street. By 1948, 2,716 associations were affiliated with it.

The Rural Nursing Association founded in the

West of England by Mrs. Malleson in 1888 was the pioneer association in county nursing. A County Nursing Association was started in Hampshire in 1891 and in Lincolnshire in 1894.

In the beginning district nursing was organized entirely by voluntary and benevolent bodies. At a later period local authorities sometimes paid for the nurses' services, and when the National Health Service was introduced in 1948, they took over the responsibility for providing district nursing services. In London today the London County Council provides much of the money needed for district nursing, but the running and co-ordination of the whole service remains in the hands of a voluntary body—the Central Council for District Nursing.

DISTRICT NURSING ABROAD

In Canada the Victorian Order of Nurses (V.O.N.) was started in 1897 by the Countess Ishbel Aberdeen, wife of the Governor-General. The nurses wore a uniform similar to that of their British colleagues, with the Queen's badge.

An Act of 1909 empowered the New Zealand Hospital Boards to spend money on nursing outside the hospitals, particularly in isolated places.

In Australia the 'Bush Nursing Association' was formed in 1911.

In 1946 the Greek War Relief Association of the United States of America agreed to train fifty Greek girls in England before starting a district nursing service in Greece.

In America Lillian Wald in 1893 established the

first nurses' settlement in New York, which from modest beginnings grew into the 'Henry Street Visiting Nurses'—the present-day 'Visiting Nurse Service of New York'.

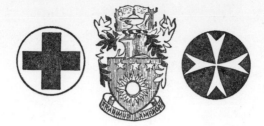

11

Nursing Councils, Colleges, and State Registration

Nurses were the first professional women to form an international association. In 1899, at a meeting of the Matrons' Council of Great Britain and Ireland, a former matron of St. Bartholomew's Hospital, Mrs. Bedford Fenwick (*née* Ethel Gordon Manson), proposed the setting up of a provisional committee to consider the matter. Her suggestion was enthusiastically supported by many leading nurses from various countries, and the International Council of Nurses came into being. Its first meeting was held at Buffalo, New York, in 1901. Active membership was offered to self-governing National Nurses' Associations, and nurses in every country were urged to form a Nurses' Association in order to be in a position to apply for membership. The Council is non-political and aims at maintaining the highest standards of nursing service, nursing education, and professional ethics in the membership countries. It is in official relationship with the World Health Organization and other welfare and social bodies. It organizes quadrennial congresses at which the nurses of the world may meet to discuss professional problems. In 1957 over 3,000 nurses representing 39 countries attended the Congress held at Rome.

The headquarters of the International Council of Nurses are at present in London.

In 1916 a group of nurses in Britain founded the College of Nursing which became the Royal College of Nursing in 1939. It is a professional organization concerned with promoting the advance of nursing in all its branches. In the early days it aimed at providing a uniform standard of training and was active in the movement to secure State Registration for Nurses. It has gradually grown, and its range of activities has increased, so that it has become the largest organization of trained nurses in Britain with a membership of over 44,000 in 1958.

The Royal College of Nursing has done pioneer work in organizing post-registration courses for nurses. Gradually these have been introduced to meet the needs of different branches of nursing. Hundreds of students, many from overseas, attend a variety of courses arranged by the education department which has centres in London, Edinburgh, Belfast, and Birmingham. Many are whole-time students preparing for additional qualifications in various branches of nursing, such as Nursing Administration, Sister Tutor Diploma, Health Visiting, Occupational Health Nursing, and Ward Sisters' Training.

Nursing Councils, Colleges and State Registration

State Registration was for some years a controversial subject in many countries. New Zealand was the first country to pass a Nurses Registration Act in 1901. Although nursing legislation was recommended by many nurses and their organizations in the United Kingdom, it was not until 1919 that the first Nurses Act was passed (see p. 54). The Nurses Act 1943 gave recognition to a second grade of nurse, laying down conditions of training and enrolment, and also made provision for the registration of qualified nurse tutors.

Expansion of training facilities to keep pace with the widening field of nursing has been catered for in the Nurses Act of 1949. Provision was made for the approval of experimental schemes of training, many of which have since been arranged. An example is one scheme of integrated training in general nursing, midwifery, and health visiting, another includes district nursing.

Progress and change in nursing have been noticeable in recent years. Rapid advances in surgery and medical practice have enabled increasing numbers of patients to be treated and have made additional claims on nurses. Acute nursing is often highly complex, being more scientific and technical than in former days. Since the introduction of the National Health Service and improvements in conditions for nurses, their numbers have increased, yet in spite of a recruitment for training of over 20,000 each year in England and Wales, there is an overall shortage.

Nursing, however, continues to be attractive to young people, and there is a vast field of work open to those who qualify. The figures given by the Ministry of Health show that over 50,000 qualified nurses were engaged in whole-time nursing in the hospital service in England and Wales in 1957, and a considerably smaller number were employed in home nursing, maternity and child-welfare work, school nursing, and health visiting.

As the concept of nursing has widened to include preventive work, training has been given to enable nurses to be health teachers, to work in clinics, schools, in the homes, and in industry.

A competent Nursing Service is vital to the success of the health and social services of any country. Further developments are dependent upon the maintenance of a progressive and adaptable nursing profession geared to meet the challenge of this changing age.

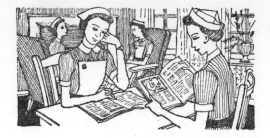

12

Nursing Journals

It is difficult for professional men and women to do their jobs properly without the aid of specialist journals. You are fortunate in having many fine periodicals at your service. In what ways does a journal help you? First and foremost it gives you news of the nursing world. There are all too few opportunities for you to meet your colleagues from overseas, and even from different parts of the country, and when personal contact is impossible, a good magazine provides the best means of keeping in touch. You can keep abreast of all legislation affecting your profession and of the recommendations made by official organizations. Articles and annotations will keep you informed of advances in the various branches of medicine, so that you will have at least a nodding acquaintance with procedures which have not so far come within your own experience.

Many nurses naturally look for news of former colleagues or for items relating to the training school or hospital where their nursing education began.

Those working in remote spots, and particularly in distant lands, have special need of contact with their professional sisters, for not only are they most likely to benefit from the practical notes on new procedures, but for them it is doubly important to be reminded that physical isolation does not cut them off from those at home.

Last, but not least, your nursing journal will help you find a suitable post.

In Great Britain the pioneers of the nursing movement were quick to appreciate the need for a professional magazine. The *Nursing Record*, 'a journal for nurses, and a chronicle of hospital and institution news', began on April 5th, 1888, and in 1893 was taken over by Mrs. Bedford Fenwick, who edited it until her death in 1947. It was due largely to her enthusiasm, inspiration, and energy that the journal increased in size and in importance when it appeared under the new name, the *British Journal of Nursing*, in 1902. For many years the official journal of the British Nurses' Association, the Matrons' Council, and the British College of Nursing, it ceased publication in April 1956.

The *Nursing Mirror* also dates from 1888 and, before assuming a separate existence, formed part of *The Hospital*. The *Nursing Times*, the official organ of the Royal College of Nursing, was founded in 1905.

All these journals may be described as almost unique in being weekly publications.

The year 1888 was important to American nurses as well as to their British colleagues, for their first national nursing periodical, *The Trained Nurse and*

Hospital Review, was started in that year. During its first decade it absorbed a number of other journals. The *American Journal of Nursing*, founded in 1900, is the official organ of the American Nurses' Association, formerly known by the somewhat cumbersome name 'Nurses Associated Alumnae of the United States and Canada'.

In 1940 *Nursing Notes and Midwives' Chronicle*, representing the Midwives' Institute, the Association for Promoting the Training of Midwives, the Colonial Nursing Association, etc., changed its title to the *Midwives' Chronicle and Nursing Notes*.

Most European countries have one or more nursing journals, the majority dating from the first decade of this century. In the international sphere there is the *International Nursing Review*, published by the International Council of Nurses.

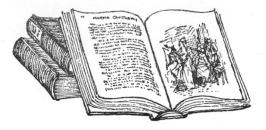

APPENDIX

The Nurse in Literature

In view of the universality of nursing it is not surprising that allusions to it occur in many branches of literature—histories, books of travel, essays, poems, and novels.

As several of the early chronicles which provide valuable source material for medieval history were written in monasteries or convents, their compilers were able to relate something of the nursing activities of the religious communities. Numerous early romances in prose and verse told of deeds enacted in the age of chivalry, and in later years such works as Tennyson's *The Idylls of the King* recalled the old stories of knighthood. In *Lancelot and Elaine* we read how the maiden nursed the wounded knight:

> *... and every day she tended him,*
> *And likewise many a night: and Lancelot*
> *Would, tho' he call'd his wound a little hurt*
> *Whereof he should be quickly whole, at times*
> *Brain-feverous in his heat and agony, seem*

Uncourteous, even he: but the meek maid
Sweetly forbore him ever, being to him
Meeker than any child to a rough nurse,
Milder than any mother to a sick child,
And never woman yet, since man's first fall,
Did kindlier unto man . . .

In the tenth canto of *The Faerie Queene* Edmund Spenser wrote of a 'holy Hospitall', and of the duties performed by the various brethren:

The fift had charge sicke persons to attend,
And comfort those, in point of death which lay. . .

Charles Kingsley's *The Saint's Tragedy* was published in the form of a poetic drama, but the story which it tells of St. Elizabeth of Hungary was originally written as a prose history and intended 'as a gift book to his wife on his marriage-day, if that day should ever come'. He says of St. Elizabeth caring for the poor:

'Does she not tend them from the cradle, nurse them, kiss their sores, feed them, bathe them, with her own hands, clothe them, living and dead, with garments. . . . Are not the hospices which she has founded in divers towns, the wonder of Germany?'

In 1815, the year of Waterloo, Robert Southey made a journey through the Low Countries, which he described in his *Journal of a Tour in the Netherlands in the Autumn of* 1815. The following is one of the many interesting passages contained in the work: 'there are about 6000 Beguines in Brabant and Flanders. . . . They receive the sick who come to them for succour, and they support as well as attend them as long as the case requires; they go out also to nurse the sick. . . . The dress of the Beguines is not inconvenient, but it is abominably ugly, as the habits of every female order are, I believe, without exception.'

Daniel Defoe achieved immortality with *Robinson Crusoe*, but among other books to his credit are many political satires and the remarkable *A Journal of the Plague Year*. The work has never been surpassed for its representation of the horror which the pestilence brought to seventeenth-century London. This macabre passage reminds us of the days when the name of nurse was more of a reproach than anything else:

'We had at this time a great many frightful stories told us of nurses and watchmen who looked after the dying people; that is to say, hired nurses, who attended infected people, using them barbarously, starving them, smothering them, or by other wicked means, hastening their end. . . .'

Louisa M. Alcott's *Little Women* was one of the most popular books with young readers of previous generations. Her book *Hospital Sketches and Companion Fireside Stories*, though less known, contains interesting accounts of her experiences as a nurse during the American Civil War. In one part she gives a humorous, but true-to-life description of how 'Nurse Periwinkle' (herself) faced up to her first nursing experience:

' "They've come! they've come! hurry up, ladies —You're wanted."

' "Who have come? The rebels?"

'This sudden summons in the gray dawn was some-

what startling to a three days' nurse like myself . . .
my room-mate took it more coolly, and, as she began
a rapid toilet . . . answered . . . it's the wounded from
Fredericksburg. . . .

'Presently the wounded were brought in and
"Nurse Periwinkle" was told: "Come my dear, begin
to wash as fast as you can. Tell them to take off
socks, coats and shirts. Scrub them well, put on
clean shirts, and the attendants will finish them off,
and lay them in bed."

'If she had requested me to shave them all, or
dance a hornpipe on the stove funnel, I should have
been less staggered; but to scrub some dozen lords
of creation at a moment's notice, was really—
really— . . . I drowned my scruples in my wash-
bowl, clutched my soap manfully, and assuming a
business-like air, made a dab at the first dirty specimen I saw. . . .'

Henry Wadsworth Longfellow's famous narrative
poem in hexameters, *Evangeline*, *A Tale of Arcadie*,
tells of the separation of Evangeline and Gabriel on
their wedding day when the French settlers were
moved from Nova Scotia by the British in 1755.
After Evangeline has searched in vain for years she
finds Gabriel, now an old and dying man, in the
Philadelphia Almshouse (now the Philadelphia
General Hospital), which she had been visiting as a
Sister of Mercy:

*And, with light in her looks, she entered the chambers
of sickness.*
*Noiselessly moved about the assiduous, careful atten-
dants,*

Appendix: The Nurse in Literature

*Moistening the feverish lip and the aching brows,
and in silence
Closing the sightless eyes of the dead.*

A cousin of Katherine Mansfield, the Australian-born Countess von Arnim was living on her husband's estate in East Prussia when she wrote anonymously the gently satirical *Elizabeth and Her German Garden*, 1898. Her husband whom she calls the 'Man of Wrath' gives vent to his feelings on the subject of private nurses:

'Gentleness and tact! I have never found those qualities in the professional nurse. According to my experience she is a disagreeable person who finds in private nursing exquisite opportunities for asserting her superiority over ordinary and prostrate mankind. I know of no more humiliating position for a man than to be in bed having his feverish brow soothed by a sprucely dressed strange woman, bristling with starch and spotlessness. He would give one-half his income for his clothes and the other half if she would leave him alone. . . . To the unimaginative, the professional nurse appears merely as an extremely self-confident woman, wisely concerned, first of all, in her personal comfort, much given to complain about her food and possessing an extraordinary capacity for fancying herself slighted or not regarded as the superior being she knows herself to be.'

It is strange that probably the best known representation of the nurse in fiction is the one least worthy of that honour. Mrs. Gamp, immortalized in Charles Dickens's *Martin Chuzzlewit*, was everything that a good nurse ought not to be, but even this harridan served a useful purpose. Like so many Dickens's characters she is more familiar than many a real person, and her shortcomings brought home to thousands the need for organization of the nursing profession.

Francis Brett Young was one of the many 'truants' from medicine who won fame as a novelist. In *Dr. Bradley Remembers* there is an interesting passage on the changes in the type of women enrolling as nurses at the turn of the century. The doctor in the story qualified in 1887, and the following scene is a description of his return to the hospital in 1905:

'He met several nurses who looked at him curiously and lowered their eyes. They were different, he thought, from the homely old bodies he used to know: younger, prettier, smarter. One would have guessed, at a glance, they were "Ladies".'

William Ernest Henley is best remembered for his poem *Invictus* with the stirring lines:

> *It matters not how strait the gate,*
> *How charged with punishments the scroll,*
> *I am the master of my fate:*
> *I am the captain of my soul.*

Henley had lost one leg through tuberculosus infection in childhood and was near to losing the other when he sought out Joseph (later Lord) Lister at the Edinburgh Infirmary. He was a patient in the Infirmary for two years and still had his leg when he was discharged. His verses 'In Hospital' were first published in the *Cornhill Magazine* in 1876. Apart from the famous tribute to 'The Chief' (Lister), Henley has given us a remarkable picture of the

'Staff-Nurse: Old Style' (Mrs. Porter) who had nursed under the great surgeon James Syme, Lister's father-in-law:

> *These thirty years she has been nursing here,*
> *Some of them under Syme, her hero still.*
> *Much is she worth, and even more is made of her.*
> *Patients and students hold her very dear.*
> *The doctors love her, tease her, use her skill.*
> *They say 'The Chief' himself is half-afraid of her.*

Some unpublished poems from the 'In Hospital' series were printed in the *Bulletin of the Institute of the History of Medicine*, Baltimore, 1936, 4, 231–41. Among them is one entitled 'Staff Nurse—New Style'. A note explains that this was deleted in the first corrected proof for the *Cornhill Magazine* by Henley himself. It affords an amusing contrast to the lines on Mrs. Porter:

> *Nurse mine—my nurse, yet not my nurse!*
> *You have delicious violet eyes,*
> *Your red lips rhyme a perfect verse,*
> *My dreams your outlines realize.*
>
> *I wish your heart were quite perverse,*
> *Your little head not quite so wise;*
> *The comedy we now rehearse*
> *Might end in truly tragic wise.*
>
> *I would that we might dare and do*
> *The deed we hardly dare to dream,*
> *The deed so far from you and me!*

Appendix: The Nurse in Literature

O me! To wrest a proof from you!
The one I need to swear supreme
Your dainty amiability.

In Thackeray's novel *The Adventures of Philip* one of the principal characters is the 'Little Sister' (Mrs. Brandon). When a girl, she was tricked into a bogus marriage and, after being deserted by her 'husband', was befriended by Dr. Goodenough, who helped her to become a nurse. Later in the story she manages to circumvent the knavery of the scoundrelly Rev. Hunt. Hunt has been drinking and, as he approaches her, she flings back a cupboard door and the key strikes his head, causing him to collapse in a chair. The 'Little Sister' remembers that in the cupboard is a bottle containing chloroform: 'In the cupboard was that bottle which she had received from America not long since; and about which she had talked with Goodenough on that very day. It had been used twice or thrice by his direction, by hospital surgeons, and under her eye.' Pouring some chloroform on a handkerchief, she approaches the injured man: 'Here, let me bathe you! Smell this. It will—it will do you —good—it will— it will, indeed! The handkerchief was over his face. Bewildered by drink before, the fumes of the liquor which he was absorbing served almost instantly to overcome him. He struggled for a moment or two.' While reassuring him, 'She squeezed more of the liquor from the bottle on to the handkerchief. In a minute Hunt was quite inanimate.'

It would seem that in using the words 'Received from America not long since', Thackeray was confusing ether and chloroform. Ether anaesthesia was

114

first employed in America by Crawford Williamson Long in 1842 and by William Thomas Green Morton in 1846. This is not the place to consider the various priority claims which make this story so intriguing and so sordid. The use of chloroform as an anaesthetic was discovered by Sir James Young Simpson in 1847. Incidentally, the extract from Thackeray is probably one of the earliest references to the use of chloroform in rendering a person insensible for other than purely medical reasons.

In Sinclair Lewis's novel *Martin Arrowsmith* we encounter a not uncommon 'misdemeanor' on the part of a nurse. During his medical studies Arrowsmith meets Leora, the nurse who becomes his wife. They have an evening out with another couple, and Leora is late back at the nurses' quarters: 'Oh, I don't care, I'll slip in through a window. If you're there in the morning, the Old Cat can't prove you got in late.'

Florence Nightingale's unique position in nursing history and the strength of her personality are reflected in the vast amount of literature devoted to her. Various aspects of her career have been presented in dramatic form, the best play, perhaps, being *The Lady with a Lamp* by Reginald Berkeley (1929).

Most people regarded the execution of Nurse Edith Cavell during the 1914–18 war as an atrocity made all the more shocking by the nature of her calling. In extenuation of the German action it has been argued that, by helping Belgians to reach the front and in aiding British troops to cross the frontier, she relinquished all right to the protection afforded to nurses. A play about this gallant woman was written by C. E. Bechhofer Roberts and C. S. Forester and produced in 1934.

In this selection from a wide range of literature an attempt has been made to give some idea of the interesting items of nursing history which are sometimes found in the most unlikely places. It has been impossible to refer to more than a fraction of the many works of fiction in which nurses are among the principal characters. There is no collection of references to nurses and nursing in general literature, while medical men have compiled several anthologies of items referring to their profession, which have been found in the course of leisure reading. Because such passages are of great historic interest and throw considerable light on conditions prevailing in days gone by, it would be a rewarding hobby for anyone who took the trouble to record all items of nursing interest encountered in novels, plays, poetry, essays, or other non-professional literature.

Index

Index

Index

Malleson, Mrs., founds Rural Nursing Association, 97–8
Manson, Ethel Gordon, *see* Fenwick, Mrs. Bedford
Margaret, Princess, 48
Martin Arrowsmith, 115
Martin Chuzzlewit, 111
Medical Record, New York, 75
Metropolitan and National Nursing Association, foundation, 96
Mikulicz-Radecki, Johann von, uses thread gloves when operating, 77
Military Medal, instituted, 59
 award to nurses, 60
Milnes, Richard Monckton, proposes to Florence Nightingale, 33
Midwives' Chronicle and Nursing Notes, 106
Monasteries, Dissolution of, 27–28
Monte Cassino, monastery, 24
Moore, Sir Norman, 52 fn., 65
Morris, Robert Tuttle, on gloves for surgeons, 75
Morton, William Thomas Green, 115
Moses, 14

National Birthday Trust, 97
New Zealand, passes Nurses' Registration Act, 102
Nightingale, Florence, 12, 47
 birth, 31
 seeks permission to nurse at Salisbury, 32
 hears of Pastor Fliedner, 32
 rejects proposal of marriage, 33
 illness, 33
 at Kaiserswerth, 33
 at convent school in Rome, 34
 works with Sisters of Saint Vincent de Paul, Paris, 34
 superintendent, Establishment for Gentlewomen during Illness, 34
 at Middlesex Hospital, 34
 at Scutari, 36–7
 system of training nurses, 38
 against registration, 38
 illness, Sir Zachary Cope on, 39
 death, 39
 on Army Medical Services reform, 39–40
 Notes on Nursing, 38
 pioneer work in statistics, 40
 suggestions for district nursing, 96
 and Queen Victoria Jubilee Institute for Nurses, 97
Nightingale, family, 32
 Fund, 37
 Nurses, uniform, 67–8
 Parthenope, 32–3
 School, 37
Nitrofurazone, introduced, 92
Nottingham General Hospital, nurses' salaries, 57
 nurses' beer allowance, 71
Nurses Act, 1919, 54
 1949, 102
Nurses Associated Alumnae of the United States and Canada, 106

121

Index

Index